GOOD CARE LEADERSHIP

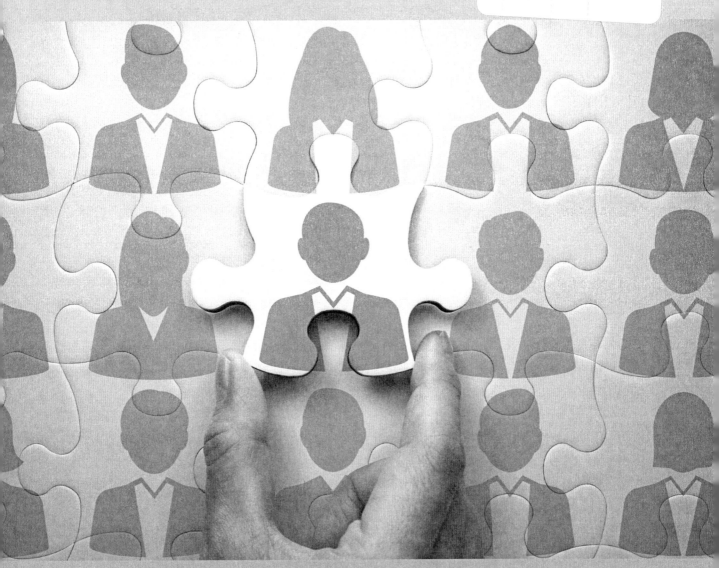

A leadership development manual for frontline health and care staff

Paul Whitby

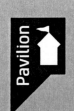

Good Care Leadership

Published by:
Pavilion Publishing and Media Ltd
Blue Sky Offices
25 Cecil Pashley Way
Shoreham by Sea
West Sussex
BN43 5FF
UK

Tel: 01273 434 943
Email: info@pavpub.com
Web: www.pavpub.com

Published 2020

A catalogue record for this book is available from the British Library.

ISBN: 978-1-913414-61-0

Pavilion Publishing and Media is a leading publisher of books, training materials and digital content in mental health, social care and allied fields. Pavilion and its imprints offer must-have knowledge and innovative learning solutions underpinned by sound research and professional values.

Author: Paul Whitby
Editor: Jo Hathaway
Cover design: Emma Dawe, Pavilion Publishing and Media
Page layout and typesetting: Phil Morash, Pavilion Publishing and Media
Printing: Ashford Press

Contents

All the resources for this training can be downloaded at
www.pavpub.com/good-care-leadership-resources

About the author

Paul Whitby is a chartered clinical psychologist and formerly a charge nurse. He has spent the majority of his career working with older adults and people with learning disabilities. He is currently a freelance trainer and is a trustee of Alzheimer's Support Wiltshire.

Acknowledgements

I am grateful to the huge number of excellent health and care professionals who, by their examples, have informed the content of this course. There are too many to mention every one individually, stretching back over a career of more than 40 years. However, I am particularly indebted to helpful conversations with Susanna Lawrence, Ray Field and Christine Voce. I hope I have properly understood their ideas and I take full responsibility for any errors or omissions.

Introduction

'Men make their own history, but they do not make it as they please; they do not make it under self-selected circumstances, but under circumstances existing already, given and transmitted from the past.'

Karl Marx

The need for leadership at the frontline of care

Jo was visiting her elderly mother in hospital and was shocked with what she found. She wrote an account of her experiences that were later published by the Patients Association (2011). This account runs to four pages and details many examples of what Jo considered poor care, including neglect of hydration, poor communication, impertinence and the loud playing of Radio 1 on an older persons' ward.

> 'The ward gave me the impression of being a chaotic place, with bells left unanswered, and staff did not introduce themselves to patients, often the elderly patients were addressed in what I consider to be the most impertinent manner by the young members of staff.'

My first impression on reading this was, 'How is it that nurses (of all people) sometimes come to be associated with poor care and neglect of vulnerable people, and sometimes even abuse? How is it that you can take a group of well-intentioned, well-trained people, put them together on a ward and get such poor outcomes?'

But then in the middle of this account I read…

> 'On Sunday the 20th of February a different sister was in charge, and the ward felt like a different place. Bells were answered promptly, staff voices seemed lower and the contact with patients felt so much better… this particular nurses [sic] skills at running a ward were exceptional. The ward was a better place when she was around."

From *We've been listening, have you been learning?*, Harrow: Patients Association, 2011, pp15–18

My reaction was that there is some hope here. Despite everything, good care is possible.

In many ways these brief quotes from Jo's account of her experience as a visitor on the ward encapsulate what this course is all about.

As you may imagine, Jo's longer account gives more details of how the care that this lady's mother received was far from perfect. This is, rather sadly, what many people have come to expect. Not as a rule, not in every case, but poor care for vulnerable people – that is, people with learning disabilities, people with chronic mental health problems and older people – happens often enough that it is no longer a surprise, but it is always a disappointment. The picture drawn is familiar: an overstretched and demoralised workforce, a group of patients with multiple and chronic disorders, both groups undervalued by the system that seems to reserve its highest regard for 'fancy', acute medical care.

And yet, and this is a very big 'yet', into this unpromising environment comes a single person in a position of authority who ensures, through her leadership skills, that the whole atmosphere of the place becomes positive and the ward becomes *a better place*. We do not know for certain, but it appears that this sister did not have too much difficulty persuading the rest of the ward staff to raise their performance, to answer bells promptly, to lower their voices and improve their contact with the patients. These were the same people who had been under-performing on the earlier days. Given the right leader, the poor performance of the entire ward staff was turned around instantaneously.

This brief anecdote illustrates the major themes that will be covered in this book:

▶ Poor care is associated with poor leadership at the level of the ward or the care home. Good leadership at this level is essential for good care.

▶ Each ward or care home has a 'culture', but that culture can vary greatly according to who is on duty and, critically, who is in charge of the shift.

▶ The person in charge at the caring frontline is absolutely key in determining this culture. No matter how much we may be buffeted by events and circumstances, by pressures of work or staffing shortages, to an extent these people can 'make their own weather'.

▶ One very practical way to improve care is to develop leadership skills in relatively junior staff. By this I mean those staff at the front-line level, the person present and in charge.

▶ Everybody has the potential to be a leader. Some are naturals and others need a little coaching. But the basics for frontline leadership are common to all clinical staff. These are the topics addressed in the first four sessions of this training course – Confidence and Competence, Values, The Use of Authority, and Motivating Others.

▶ The leader, whether they are matron, sister or staff nurse, or even OT, social worker, or doctor, depends upon his or her junior staff. *The people who know how to improve care on wards and in care homes are already working there.* The good leader will bring out all the potential for good care from their staff, especially the poor performers.

Anybody who has worked on wards and in care homes will already know much of this. They will probably have met a person like the sister mentioned above and consequently they already know what to do!

These topics will be addressed on this course with the final session looking at how to put them ideas into action. Knowledge about leadership is worth nothing if it is not acted upon.

I hope that it will be clear throughout this book that I have the greatest respect and admiration for the members of all the caring professions. It has been my privilege to work alongside these people for most of my life. Of course some are better at their jobs than others, but whatever human failings, weaknesses and blemishes I have both witnessed and demonstrated personally, the overwhelming experience has been a positive one: of people who try hard, give more than could be fairly expected and who return to the frontline of care, day after day, year after year, knowing they can rarely 'succeed' but determined to do the best that they can.

This course is hugely optimistic and it is this way because of my experiences and the people I have met. It is always preferable to light a candle than to curse the darkness. There may well be a lot of darkness, but there are also an awful lot of candles. If just half of the time spent analysing what went wrong at Stafford Hospital, for example, had been spent on analysing how people like the Sister mentioned above get it right, then we might be a lot further along the road to universal good care than we are now. There is a well-established school of psychotherapy and coaching that states explicitly that time spent discussing the problem is time wasted. According to this method, unsurprisingly named the Solutions Focus approach, the best way forward is to spend your time thinking about and planning for solutions and improvements, looking for examples when things go well and taking small steps in the right direction. This approach is suitable for developing a whole range of personal skills and is perfectly suited for developing as a leader.

Good care requires good leadership

'Let whoever is in charge keep this simple question in her head (not, how can I always do this right thing myself, but) how can I provide for this right thing to be always done?'

Florence Nightingale

The ward sister who we noted above did not improve the care on her ward by offering personal care nursing and attending to sick individuals. She was doing something on a different plane; she was *leading*. She was organising a group of junior staff and ensuring that during her shift *'…the ward felt like a different place. Bells were answered promptly, staff voices seemed lower and the contact with patients felt so much better.'* She was creating the circumstances in which her staff could perform the best they knew how to and she was motivating them to do so. By doing this she raised the quality of care for all the patients on the ward. This is the challenge for all nurses and care staff in all positions of responsibility, however minor that responsibility may seem to be. Being in charge of a group of people, even for only a few hours, requires a different set of skills to those required for giving individual care. This course is all about the development of that skill set.

Health and care professionals generally enter their profession because they enjoy the individual contact and the sense of being helpful and kind to sick people. Most of their training involves learning clinical skills to provide the correct care for individuals. Yet soon after they are qualified most will be expected to take charge of a team. This is a different task and requires a new set of skills. They are moving from *doing care* to *supervising and leading a team*.

Experience shows us that it is likely that, with no significant training in leadership skills, a fair number turn out to be 'naturals'. They just take to it with ease. However, there are many others who struggle with leadership and who could do with some supportive professional development. Certainly, I was one of those. I really could have been a better staff nurse and charge nurse in so many ways if, early on, I had been introduced to the ideas that I slowly picked up over the following years. My hope is that with a bit of time devoted to following through the concepts presented in this course, all frontline care professionals and their immediate managers will be able to fulfil their potential for leading their teams even more effectively than they do now.

The danger is that, without decent leadership, care teams will underperform. Many of the pressures on frontline staff will tend to push them away from good care, towards low morale, burnout and 'care-lessness'. Good leadership is the antidote to this outcome, as has been recognised for decades. It is possible to be a good leader and provide decent care, even in difficult and unfavourable situations such as those for the Sister in the quote at the head of the chapter shows.

The real action is on the clinical frontline

When we think of important people in the health services, social services and care services we very often think of people in senior management and professional positions. However, without wishing in any way to minimise the importance of these senior people, it is worth pointing out that the less senior staff, those who are at the clinical frontline, are equally important, even though they are lower down the hierarchy and generally draw smaller salaries.

Leadership not only starts at the frontline but it is also at its *most important* there. This is where staff meet patients or residents; this is where interactions and procedures are carried out with kindness and compassion (or not); this is where the patients' fears and worries are dealt with.

Frontline leaders have daily and close contact with the staff who are providing care, and are themselves in contact with patients and relatives. If a healthcare organisation can be judged on the quality of the care that it offers then these people are absolutely crucial. It is the care staff, qualified professionals and assistants, who patients remember. It is their actions that leave a lasting impression. In very practical terms, care is not delivered by 'an organisation' or by a 'culture'; care is delivered in hundreds of interpersonal interactions between staff and patients over the duration of the patient's episode of care. The person who is in the best position to monitor and manage the staff's interactions is their frontline manager.

Frontline leaders often have very close contact with the patients and relatives on the wards and care homes they lead. Worried people will often seek out the nurse in charge, or equivalent, for reassurance or with their concerns. It is this person, the accessible face of authority, who often has the greatest impact on their experience.

Furthermore, today's frontline leaders are the senior managers of tomorrow. Time spent developing their leadership skills will not only improve their performance in their current job but will provide them with a set of experiences, knowledge and skills that they can carry with them as their career develops and as some of them move up the corporate hierarchy.

Leadership is for everyone

Given the widespread need for good leadership, it is logical to ensure that everybody gets decent leadership development opportunities. Every ward, care home, team and department needs good leadership all the time and this leadership is not to be located solely in one person or the top team. It is found all the way down the chain of command. Leadership training should be given greater priority than it has now for a far greater number of lower grade, frontline staff. This is because anybody who has any responsibility or any leadership role whatsoever at the frontline of patient care has a crucial and direct impact on the care that patients receive.

Ideally, all the qualified staff from all professions on a ward should be offered leadership training as a group. This would allow for the development of a 'critical mass' of enthusiastic leaders, for joint goals and projects to be planned, and for mutual support in difficult times.

Studies of leadership and personality have failed to find any specific personality traits that determine successful leadership performance. On the contrary, some studies conclude that good leaders often will suppress some aspects of their personality and maybe develop traits that are not naturally strong, depending upon the circumstances and the demands of the situation. Leadership, it appears, is more about acting, about behaving in response to the demands of a situation, than it is about having the 'right personality'. Leadership is about what you do and what you accomplish and consequently it is open to all.

Leadership opportunities are ever present

Leadership is not something that is exclusive to the highest grades in the health and care services. The opportunities and the need for leadership occur at all levels, and it is particularly pressing where interventions with patients are involved. Each patient, care professional and ward or care home is unique. Management cannot dictate how a nurse or a team must behave in each and every situation; there are laws, policies and guidelines to map out the territory. However, on many occasions, each day, every professional will be called upon to weigh options, set priorities and make decisions that are of vital importance to people in their care. The scope for getting things right – or not – is enormous.

A staff nurse in charge of a shift at a weekend will have to do all the management tasks, including allocating and supervising duties, ensuring all necessary procedures are performed and records are kept. She will also have duties that are more to do with leadership, such as trying to set the tone of the ward atmosphere. If we try to imagine how the ward sister at the head of the chapter would have achieved the remarkable alteration in ward culture, we might think that she would be using language that conveyed respect for her patients. She would be clear about her standards and would clearly state what was expected and what would not be tolerated. For example, she would not refer to 'the stroke in bed 4', or if one of her staff made a remark about Mrs Jones being 'demanding' she might respond with a frown and reframe this as Mrs Jones being understandably very worried about her upcoming discharge. This sister might show her values by ensuring staff get their breaks, that their efforts are noted and commented upon favourably, that unpleasant or difficult tasks are allocated fairly. Leadership is shown in the multitude of interactions that occur every day and it most certainly is not restricted to major projects or grand schemes.

Consistency, persistence and quality of small leadership actions over time are what makes a good leader.

There is a case to be made that the importance of good leadership is greatest the closer one is to face-to-face patient care, because that is where the impact of the entire organisation is felt. All the business that goes under the name of 'senior management' – the budgeting, the strategic direction, the policies, the IT systems and the like – also have an effect on patient care but it is difficult to be precise about exactly what. In contrast, we know that the behaviour of the staff who come into contact with patients and care home residents to deliver care do have a clear and measurable effect upon their well-being.

One is reminded of Peter Hyman, the former speech writer and communications director to Tony Blair, who left policy making in Downing Street to return to classroom teaching because he felt that real improvements are made, not by big gestures and policy, but by smaller things, seriously implemented over a long period of time.

The frontline is where the action is.

A simple model for frontline leadership

The model of care leadership used in this course contains four elements. A good leader will possess all of these elements to some degree because none by itself is sufficient. Some people will be stronger in one area than in others and each leader's pattern will be unique.

The constellation of four elements is:

1. Your competences and the confidence that these bring.

2. Strong personal values.

3. The appropriate use of authority, influence and power.

4. Motivating others in your team.

The model is very simple and it is also unusual. Unlike many models of leadership that describe leadership behaviour and give a 'ideal' model of what a leader should be like, this model looks for the foundation of leadership in the make-up of the individual themselves. It acknowledges that there is no single perfect way of being a leader, that people and situations are endlessly variable. What it seeks to do is to ensure that every frontline leader reaches the potential that lies within them. There is some didactic teaching on this course. There are mini-lectures to clarify some concepts and some information on power and motivation that will be new to some people. Mostly, the sessions will be spent asking the participants to reflect upon aspects of their work and themselves that are too often ignored in professional development. The final session is devoted to making a plan to put what has been learned in to action. This is important as it gives participants the opportunity to practise leadership in a conscious way, aware of what they are doing and hopefully opening up previously untried ways of behaving.

Guiding principles

1. **Respect for frontline care staff.** This whole course is based on the notion that the people best placed to improve care in hospitals and homes are already working in them. These are the people with the knowledge, skills and values who have the potential to really make things happen. Their hard work and dedication are rarely recognised. Also, they have great potential for development if only they are given the right environment to flourish.

2. **Attending to solutions and strengths** is far more helpful than focusing on weaknesses and mistakes. Frontline care professionals are always trying their best and much of the time they are doing well. Criticising them for being less than perfect is likely to lead to demoralisation and resentment. Instead, on this course we look at people's strengths and what they are doing right. Paying attention to what works and doing more of it is a very practical approach.

3. **Situations matter at least as much as personality.** While 'character' is important in caring, it is also essential that the professionals are surrounded by an environment, a 'culture', that nurtures their good practice and makes it natural for them to perform at their best. Fortunately, part of the situation is directly under the influence of frontline staff, especially the leader. This is the emotional and psychological culture. Everybody present on a ward or in a care home contributes to the culture. It is usual for the more senior staff to have the most influence but we acknowledge that junior staff can also be important influencers.

Who might benefit from this course?

In the light of the remarks above, it will be clear that this course will be of benefit to any frontline health or care professional who has a leadership or supervisory role over other staff members.

In hospitals this would include:

▶ staff nurses and midwives

▶ ward managers

▶ modern matrons

▶ associate nurses with supervisory responsibilities

▶ occupational therapists

▶ physiotherapists

▶ social workers

▶ doctors

▶ speech and language therapists

▶ clinical and health psychologists.

In care homes this would include:

▶ nurses

▶ care home managers

▶ shift leaders

▶ senior care workers

▶ Social care and social work team leaders and managers.

This training is applicable in a wide range of settings as the model of good care leadership is not specific to any particular team. For example:

▶ An NHS Trust Training Department could use it to bring staff from many wards together for a large training exercise to ensure that leadership skills are widely cultivated throughout the trust.

▶ Managers or senior carers in a care home for older people could use it to train their staff to develop their leadership potential.

▶ It could be used for in-house training in a social services learning disability day centre.

The trainer

Most of the exercises described in this training guidance are fairly straightforward and can be delivered by anyone with some experience of training, especially in running group learning exercises.

It is helpful, but not essential, that they also have experience of leadership in a caring role, in a hospital, a care home or day centre.

The apparent simplicity of the exercises should not conceal the fact that they are rooted in a lot of thinking and theory. It is suggested that anybody wishing to use this resource should familiarise themselves with most of the material referred to in the 'Theory and Evidence' section on pages 92 to 102.

Using the training resource

The training takes the form of five sessions. Most of the sessions are taken up with individual and group exercises. There is some explicit teaching in Sessions 3 and 4 concerned with clarifying concepts of power, or authority, and motivation. It is expected that most of the participants will be aware, to some extent, of the material being spoken about; the introductions or 'mini-lectures' at the beginning of each session are simply making clear the approach taken on this course. For example, we all have some knowledge of our own motivation, whether we can articulate it well or not. However, the science of motivation is quite complicated and detailed and it certainly is not necessary for care practitioners to know. The use of the terms 'Junk Food Motivation' and 'Wholesome Motivation' makes clear the significant distinction between the two major types of motivation and also shows clearly which is to be favoured.

The exercises are undertaken individually, in pairs or in groups. The intention is to stimulate discussion, to encourage people to share their own knowledge and opinions and to learn from that of others. The trainer should be competent in leading exercises and group discussions.Because all the sessions are interlinked and refer to the same underlying model of leadership, there is a considerable amount of repetition. This is intended to remind the participants of key points. Trainers should use their judgement to adjust this element depending on the time between sessions. If sessions are run closely together over just a few days then less will be needed. If there is a longer time between sessions, more repetition may be needed as a reminder of material that might otherwise have been forgotten.

The training modules

The five training sessions are interlinked; it is strongly recommended that all five are delivered as a course. Each session takes between 2.5–3 hours, so the total time required is two and a half days. There is also a need for a follow-up session for reporting on the projects that were planned in Session 5; this will need to be arranged according to local needs.

The five sessions are:

Session 1: Confidence and Competence – a series of exercises designed to focus participants' attention on their skills, knowledge and accomplishments. This is designed to increase their confidence and their sense of being able to exert their influence.

Session 2: Personal Values – exercises designed to bring out the values that participants bring to their work. These are *personal* values and will be, to an extent, idiosyncratic. It is through being able to work according to our values that we gain meaning from our work.

Session 3: Use of Authority – an obligation of leadership is the exercise of power over others. This does not mean simply telling people what to do. Five forms of interpersonal power at work are explored.

Session 4: Motivating Others – This session takes much of what has been learned in the previous sessions and looks at ways that they can be applied to the team in the workplace. It also introduces the notion of belonging as important to motivation.

Session 5: Project – Putting It Into Practice – taking classroom learning to the workplace. An opportunity for participants to put the knowledge and skills learned on the course into action in a real-world setting.

Session 1: Confidence and Competence

Timing: 3 hours

Overview

Participants are provided with a view of confidence in their competence that shows it is not fixed but varies over time and from place to place. There are then a series of exercises that allow them to take a realistic and positive view of their strengths, talents and experience.

Activity	Time required
Introduction to the session	10 mins
Introduction to confidence	20 mins
Exercise 1.1: When I am more or less confident	30 mins
Exercise 1.2: My career achievements so far	20 mins
Exercise 1.3: Three challenges faced	20 mins
Exercise 1.4: A good leader I have known	30 mins
Exercise 1.5: How am I so wonderful?	40 mins
Session summary	10 mins

Materials

▶ Slides 1.1 to 1.19

▶ Handout 1.1: Discuss a time I was…

▶ Handout 1.2: What have I achieved, so far?

▶ Handout 1.3: Three challenges

▶ Handout 1.4: A good leader I have known

▶ Handout 1.5: How am I so wonderful?

▶ A1 flipchart or whiteboard

▶ pens

Introduction to the session

Timing: 10 mins

Aims

▶ To welcome the participants to the training

▶ To inform participants of the programme for the day

▶ Introductions: to find out who is in the room

Materials

▶ Slide 1.1: Welcome

▶ Slide 1.2: Programme

▶ Slide 1.3: Four components of good care leadership

Notes for the trainer

1. Show *Slide 1.1: Welcome*

▶ Welcome learners to the training day, introducing yourself and giving participants some background information about yourself as appropriate.

▶ Outline housekeeping arrangements, such as the procedure in the event of a fire, the mobile phone policy and the location of toilets etc.

▶ Invite participants to introduce themselves to the group, stating their name, a brief description of their role and what they would like to get out of the session's training.

2. Show and read out *Slide 1.2: Programme* and inform participants that there is a lot to fit in so you will need to keep to the timings listed, but that within these constraints you will welcome questions at any point in the proceedings.

3. Show *Slide 1.3: Four components of good care leadership*. Explain that each of the first four sessions in this training looks at a different one of the four components of good care leadership. All four sessions interact and overlap and all are necessary.

Introduction to confidence

Timing: 20 mins

Aims

▶ To introduce participants to the idea of 'confidence' not as a fixed attribute of a person's character but as something that varies over time and from situation to situation. Most people are neither extremely and constantly 'Confident' nor 'Unconfident' but vary somewhere in between these two extremes.

Materials

▶ Slide 1.4: Ways of viewing confidence 1

▶ Slide 1.5: Ways of viewing confidence 2

▶ Slide 1.6: False confidence and true confidence

Notes for the trainer

1. Ask the group if there is anybody present who considers themselves *very confident*. Ask the group if there is anybody present who considers themselves *very unconfident*. Ask the group if there is anybody present who is a bit in the middle.

Show **Slide 1.4: Ways of viewing confidence 1**. Explain that people sometimes view themselves (and others) as being fundamentally confident or unconfident. This view makes it seem difficult to move from unconfident to confident because it is such a big leap.

2. Show **Slide 1.5: Ways of viewing confidence 2**. Explain that another way of viewing confidence is that people fall between the two poles of a continuum, with most of us somewhere in the middle. This view makes it clear that you can move from unconfident to confident gradually, in small steps.

▶ Ask the group if anybody present is confident in some situations and unconfident in others.

▶ Ask the group if they feel that their level of confidence has changed with time.

▶ Explain that this shows that confidence is not a fixed quantity. Although some people may have a general predisposition one way or another, mostly confidence fluctuates greatly.

3. Show **Slide 1.6: False confidence and true confidence**. Explain that it is common to feel very confident at the beginning of taking up a career, starting a new job, heading a new project. Often this confidence vanishes in the face of the harsh reality of the task. This is followed by a trough of despondency. With time, and with nurturing, the person's sense of confidence recovers slowly and accurately reflects their abilities. In some circumstances it does not and the person remains lacking in confidence in the long term.

Exercise 1.1: When am I more or less confident?

Timing: 30 mins

Aims

▶ To encourage participants to reflect on their own experiences of feeling confident and of not feeling confident

▶ To consider that we all vary in our feelings of confidence and that some of this is due to the situation we are in

Materials

▶ Slide 1.7: Discuss a time I was…

▶ Handout 1.1: Discuss a time I was…

▶ flipchart or whiteboard

▶ pens

Notes for the trainer

1. Ask the participants to form into pairs.

2. Show **Slide 1.7 Discuss a time I was…** and give participants **Handout 1.1** of the same name.

Ask participants to take turns in discussing and making notes on a time they can recall when they felt a) confident and b) unconfident. These do not have to be the most extreme examples from their experience, just something they feel comfortable talking about.

Allow 10 minutes for this part of the exercise.

3. Come back together as a whole group. Go round the group one at a time. Ask the group to share one of their personal top factors for *enhancing* their confidence. Write each contribution up on the flipchart or whiteboard.

4. Once again, go round the group one at a time (maybe in reverse order this time). Ask each person to share one of their personal top factors contributing to them *lacking* confidence. Write each contribution up on the flipchart or whiteboard.

5. Discuss these contributions. None will be right or wrong but they will reflect the variety of influences on the participants' sense of confidence. Explain that the next exercise aims to influence this *sense of confidence* by focusing on their strengths, talents and competencies. If possible, identify contributions from the first part of this exercise that illustrate this. For example, when participants have said that they feel more confident when they recall previous successes, or when they think something like *"If she can do it then so can I"*.

Allow 20 minutes for this part of the exercise.

Prompts and questions

Depending on the time available ask some of the following questions:

▶ How did your feeling of being confident or not affect what you do (eg what tasks or opportunities you take on or avoid)?

▶ Which feels better, being confident or not confident?

▶ Do you think 'confidence' is a fixed personal characteristic, or is it changeable?

▶ Are you already beginning to think about how colleagues, leaders and managers affect our sense of confidence by what they do and say?

Exercise 1.2: My career achievements so far

Timing: 20 mins

Aims

▶ To enhance participants' sense of self-confidence by directing their attention to their successes and achievements

Materials

▶ Slide 1.8: What have I achieved?

▶ Handout 1.2: What have I achieved so far?

Notes for the trainer

1. Show **Slide 1.8: What have I achieved?** and give out **Handout 1.2: What have I achieved so far?**

▶ Explain that there are many different kinds of achievement at work. Some are 'big' things that go on CVs and job applications. Other achievements are smaller things that give more personal satisfaction. Encourage participants to include learning experiences and tasks completed. All of them are important and everybody will have a great number of achievements in their career so far.

▶ The task now is to work on your own to write down these work achievements. This is a private exercise so there is no need to be shy or worry that people might think you are bragging.

▶ Allow 10 minutes for this part of the exercise.

2. Call the group back together again. Do not ask for specific examples of achievements from individual participants, instead ask for general comments and feedback on the exercise.

Allow 10 minutes for this part of the exercise.

Prompts and questions

Depending on the time available ask some of the following questions:

▶ Were there any surprises? Things you had forgotten maybe?

▶ Does what counts as an 'achievement' differ from person to person?

Exercise 1.3: Three challenges faced

Timing: 20 mins

Aims

▶ To enhance participants' sense of self-confidence by directing their attention toward some difficulties that they have struggled with

Materials

▶ Slide 1.9: Three challenges

▶ Handout 1.3: Three challenges

Notes for the trainer

1. Show **Slide 1.9: Three challenges**.

▶ Explain that this exercise is to get participants to think about some significant challenges in their careers. Challenges that have been important or formative for them. Sometimes we really only know what we are capable of when we are under stress or faced with a really difficult situation. These do not have to be challenges that were entirely overcome. In fact, they may be things that continue to pose a challenge to this day.

▶ It could be a challenge that lasted a long time or it could be a challenge that came and went in an instant.

2. Give out **Handout 1.3: Three challenges**. Ask participants to consider up to three challenges they have faced and to write brief notes on each challenge. Also, ask what they learned about themselves and their capabilities from this challenge.

Note: This is a private exercise that participants are not expected to share with the group.

Allow 10 minutes for this exercise.

3. Call the group back together again. Do not ask for specific examples of achievements from individual participants, instead ask for general comments and feedback on the exercise.

Allow 10 minutes for this part of the exercise.

Prompts and questions

Depending on the time available ask some of the following questions:

▶ Were there any surprises? Things you had forgotten maybe?

▶ Did you learn much about yourself from these experiences?

Points for the trainer to cover

▶ Difficulties and challenges are inevitable at work. To find something hard does not mean you are a failure.

▶ Difficulties and challenges stretch us and help us to grow, sometimes in surprising ways.

"Ever tried? Ever failed? No matter. Try again. Fail again. Fail better."

– Samuel Beckett

Exercise 1.4: A good leader I have known

Timing: 30 mins

Aims

▶ For participants to call to mind a significant role model from their past and to consider what they have learned from this person

▶ To consider that they may be filling this role themselves in their current post

Materials

▶ Handout 1.4: A good leader I have known

▶ A1 flipchart or whiteboard

▶ pens

Notes for the trainer

1. Distribute *Handout 1.4: A good leader I have known*.

▶ Explain that this is an exercise in which participants are asked to think of a person they have met who has been a role model of leadership for them. This is an important way of learning to lead and influence others, by trying to follow the examples of people who impress us.

▶ Explain that what is being asked for is somebody who participants have met and who has been a particularly good example to them, a professional role model, as it were. You are not asking for great civic, religious, military or political leaders but for somebody who the participants have met and seen at work.

▶ Ask the participants to spend a few minutes writing some brief notes on the handout and then forming into pairs to discuss their chosen person and what it was about him or her that impressed them.

▶ Allow 10 minutes for this part of the exercise.

2. Come back together as a group. Ask for contributions from each pair. Ask each participant to suggest the one most important characteristic of the leader they have chosen. Write each idea up on the flipchart or whiteboard.

▶ Sum up by saying that much leadership is achieved by influencing others around them. Many people, especially younger or junior staff, do not feel confident about their ability to influence other people. Having met and worked with at least one person who was a good leader shows that they do actually know quite a lot about leadership and influence already. They have learned from example.

Prompts and questions

Depending on the time available ask some of the following questions:

▶ How much of their leadership behaviour was *utterly fantastic* and how much was fairly ordinary?

▶ Was this person perfect? Or did he or she show ordinary human failings?

Points for the trainer to cover

▶ There are be no right or wrong answers. People are touched in different ways. Furthermore, some attributes are more appropriate in some circumstances than others, e.g. good leadership in a casualty department may differ from good leadership in a Learning Disabilities residential care home.

▶ Try to ensure everybody contributes. Because any contribution shows that they already know a lot about good leadership. They have learned it through experience.

▶ Ask whether they would consider it possible that at work *they* are viewed as a role model by some of their junior staff or other colleagues?

Exercise 1.5: How am I so wonderful?

Timing: 40 mins

Aim

▶ To consolidate the learning in the previous three exercises by asking participants to list all their strengths and achievements that makes them so good at their jobs

▶ To focus intensely upon participants' strengths and capabilities

Materials

▶ Slide 1.10: Perfect vs Useless 1

▶ Slide 1.11: Perfect vs Useless 2

▶ Handout 1.5: How am I so wonderful?

Notes for the trainer

1. Show **Slide 1.10: Perfect vs Useless 1**.

▶ Explain that one way of viewing one's talents is to put them into two extreme and mutually exclusive categories. Occasionally, this is a useful way to view the world. For example, if you have taken your driving test you are someone who has either Passed or Failed. However, most of the time it can make a lot of sense to regard such characteristics as a continuum, a scale from one extreme to the other with lots of shades of grey in the middle.

2. Show **Slide 1.11: Perfect vs Useless 2**.

▶ Explain that this slide shows how we can understand ourselves, and others, as being somewhere between the extremes. The instructions for this exercise are a little unusual so ask the group to pay particular attention.

3. Give out **Handout 1.5: How am I so wonderful?**

▶ Firstly, ask the group individually to assign themselves a score on their performance as a professional between zero – 'Completely useless', and 10 – 'Practically perfect'. (You should say that nobody who is still in employment is completely useless.) Allow two minutes for this part of the exercise.

Secondly, ask the group to form in to pairs and to discuss the reasons for this score. For the purposes of this exercise the only reasons you want them to discuss are:

▶ "What is it about you that gives you a score of 'x' rather than 'x minus 1' or 'x minus 2'?"

So, for example, if you have assigned yourself a score of 5, what is it about you that gives you this score of 5 rather than a 4 or a 3? What talents, knowledge and skills do you have, what do you do, what is in your heart that makes you a 5 rather than a 4 or a 3?

The purpose of this exercise is to focus participants' minds on their strengths. Explain that there may be a tendency to talk about why you are 'only a 5' and all the reasons why you are not a 6 or a 7 or even higher. This exercise is different. It may feel a little strange and even uncomfortable. Nonetheless, go ahead and give it a go, talk about your strengths and competencies.

4. Explain that this is an exercise intended to bring together a lot of what has been discussed in the previous exercises. You can encourage participants to put down qualities or experiences or motivations that they have already talked about or written down. Also, they should feel free to introduce new material if they wish.

Allow 20 minutes for this part of the exercise.

5. Go round the pairs and ensure everybody has a full understanding of the instructions. Encourage participants to focus on their strengths and not to be lured into "Why I am not better than a 5" talk. Make sure both members of the pair have a roughly equal time to talk.

Bring the group back together and ask for feedback.

Prompts and questions

Depending on the time available, ask some of the following questions:

▶ How did it feel to talk about why you are so good?

▶ Are you ever asked by their managers or leaders to talk about how good you are?

▶ What feelings come with talking about how good you are?

▶ What feelings come with talking about how useless you are?

Points for the trainer to cover

You may need to say that the number each person assigns themselves has meaning only for them. These numbers do not have any meaning for comparing one person against another. A person who ranks themselves an 8 is not necessarily a better professional than one who ranks herself as a 5. All it means is that she has a different understanding of her qualities and her situation from the person who gave herself a 5.

Session summary

Timing: 10 mins

Aims

▶ To summarise and remind participants of the session's content and their contributions

▶ To point out how the material produced by them fits together into the concept of Confidence and Competence and this in turn fits in with the whole Good Care Leadership course

Materials

▶ Slide 1.12: Confidence in my competence: Part of leadership

▶ Slide 1.13: Confidence in my competence: A continuum

▶ Slide 1.14: Confidence in my competence: False confidence

▶ Slide 1.15: Confidence in my competence: Confidence varies

▶ Slide 1.16: Confidence in my competence: Your achievements

▶ Slide 1.17: Confidence in my competence: Three challenges

▶ Slide 1.18: Confidence in my competence: A good leader

▶ Slide 1.19: Confidence in my competence: How am I so wonderful?

Notes for the trainer

Introduce this last section by saying that this is a quick reminder of the contents of the session and how all parts relate to each other.

1. Show *Slide 1.12: Confidence in my competence: Parts of leadership*. Explain confidence in oneself is an important part of being a frontline leader and influencer. There is little use in being the best nurse/HCA/physiotherapist/doctor in the world if you do not have the confidence to say your piece at times when you feel things could be done better.

2. Show *Slide 1.13: Confidence in my competence: A continuum* – a reminder that 'confidence' is not a single property you either have or do not have, but a continuum. You may be 'a bit confident' or maybe 'quite a lot confident', somewhere on this line.

3. Show *Slide 1.14: Confidence in my competence: False confidence*. False confidence is common and is often seen at the beginning of a career, a job or a project. It is often followed by a crash. Hopefully, it is then followed by a slower rise in true confidence that grows with time and experience.

4. Show *Slide 1.15: Confidence in my competence: Confidence varies*. Confidence also varies from time to time and from situation to situation. Some of this will

depend on you and some of it will depend on the situation you are in and the people around you. You discussed some of the factors that have affected you in the past.

5. Show **Slide 1.16: Confidence in my competence: Your achievements**. You then discussed some of your achievements, in the widest possible sense.

6. Show **Slide 1.17: Confidence in my competence: Three challenges** – you talked about three challenges that have been significant to you in your career.

7. Show **Slide 1.18: Confidence in my competence: A good leader**. You then spent some time thinking about a role model, a good leader that you have known and considered what you might have learned from them

8. Show **Slide 1.19: Confidence in my competence: How am I so wonderful?** Finally, summing up and bringing this all together, you did an exercise looking at all these aspects of your competence and how you feel about your brilliance as a professional.

Thank the group for their participation and their contributions. Ask if there are any questions.

Session 2: Personal Values

Timing: 3 hours

Overview

This session will assist participants in articulating the values that brought them into the caring professions in the first place and reflecting on how these values have developed during their career. This may also serve as a reminder of these values. There is also an opportunity to discuss the complementary nature of personal and professional values.

Activity	Time required
Introduction to the session	10 mins
Introduction to personal values	20 mins
Exercise 2.1: Writing my own retirement speech	45mins
Exercise 2.2: Choosing values from the list	45 mins
Exercise 2.3: Realising values in my current work	45mins
Session summary	15 mins

Materials

▶ Slides 2.1 to 2.20

▶ Handout 2.1: Your own retirement speech

▶ Handout 2.2: Choosing your own values

▶ Handout 2.3a: Values in your daily work

▶ Handout 2.3b: Values in your daily work

Introduction to the session

Timing: 10 mins

Aim

▶ To welcome participants to the session and to inform them of the programme for the day

Materials

▶ Slide 2.1: Welcome

▶ Slide 2.2: Programme

▶ Slide 2.3: Four components of good care leadership

Notes for the trainer

1. Show *Slide 2.1: Welcome*

▶ Welcome the learners back to this next session.

▶ Remind learners of housekeeping arrangements as appropriate.

2. Show *Slide 2.2: Programme*. Tell participants that there is a lot to fit in so you will need to keep to the timings listed, but that within these constraints you will welcome questions at any point in the proceedings.

3. Show *Slide 2.3: Four components of good care leadership*. Explain that this is the second of four sessions in this training looking at a different one of the four components of good care leadership. All four sessions interact and overlap and all are necessary.

Introduction to values

Timing: 20 mins

Aim

▶ To introduce the concept of personal values, to explain their nature and to distinguish them from professional values

▶ To emphasise the importance of values as motivators and guides to performance in health and care work

▶ To remind participants of values that they all have; these values may be more or less clearly articulated, more or less firmly held

Materials

▶ Slides 2.4 to 2.10: Personal values 1

▶ Slide 2.11: Personal values 2

▶ A1 flipchart or whiteboard

▶ pens

Instructions

1. Show **Slides 2.4 to 2.11: Personal values (1)** and **2.12: Personal values (2)**.

Reveal **Slides 2.4 to 2.10** one bulleted sentence at a time, until you arrive at **Slide 2.11** which puts all the points together in order. Use the following commentary:

a) Give meaning to our work

Personal values are what give meaning to our everyday working lives. They do not describe *what* we do, instead they describe *why* we do it. Personal values are what drive us to come to work day after day, to continue in a job that is sometimes difficult and sometimes thankless. They are what the whole of your work is all about and in the long run it is the values that you live by that will give your career in the health and care services some meaning.

b) Are a constant guide for our behaviour – *"Am I on the right track?"* (and the track is not always straight)

On a day-to-day basis our values let us know that we are doing the right thing. Most of the time they give us guidance about how to behave in any situation. When we act against our values we feel uncomfortable. This is not to say that we can always act in a way that is true to our values. Sometimes life puts immovable obstacles in our path and we need to divert a bit to get around. However, at some point we can pick up the right direction again and start acting in accordance with our values.

c) Are associated with strong feelings – including uncomfortable feelings

Personal values are not cool and rational, they are filled with strong emotions. When we act according to our values, even if it is difficult to do so, we have a sense of vitality, well-being and satisfaction. When we act against our values we feel uncomfortable, troubled even. It is sometimes the case that this discomfort is what lets us know most strongly what our values are and how we need to be changing direction in life.

This does not mean that values are the same as feelings and certainly not the same as feeling good. Sometimes acting in accordance with your values will be quite an uncomfortable choice to make.

d) Do not need to be reasoned, they are 'just there'

Personal values are a bit like personal taste. They exist beyond reason and cannot be proven to be right or wrong. Just as you cannot persuade a person who does not like peanut butter that they are wrong and ought to like peanut butter, you cannot persuade somebody that they ought to have the value of, for example, fairness. Values tend to be just there, taken for granted, part of the person you are.

This does not mean that they are inflexible. As you grow and gain experience some of your values will possibly change or some will come to seem more important and others less important.

Also, values are not arbitrary. Especially in the health and social care services we tend to find that many people have similar values. They will never be exactly the same, every person is an individual after all. But the values they have will tend to be around cure, care and support for vulnerable individuals.

e) Are never fully achieved, are constantly in action

Personal values can never be fully achieved, they can only be lived out constantly through your actions. They are not like goals that can be reached. If you have a value of fairness then there will never be a time when you have achieved 'fairness' and can stop and put that value aside. To have a value of fairness means to try to put that value into action every time that it is called for.

▶ Ask the participants for an example of a goal that has recently been set at work.

▶ Write this up on the flipchart or whiteboard, marked clearly as a goal.

▶ Then ask if they can think of the values that were behind that goal.

▶ Write these up on the flipchart or whiteboard, clearly marked as values.

▶ So, values are associated with goals, but they are different from goals. The values will remain even when the goals are achieved.

f) Indicate the direction of travel rather than the destination

Another way of thinking of this is that values are more like a direction that you wish to travel in rather than the destination. Say you wish to travel east, you will follow a compass direction for east. If you meet an obstacle like a mountain or a river you will have to abandon your pure east direction to get around that obstacle and then you will be able to take up travelling east once more. But you will never achieve "east".

This does not mean that there is no reward or satisfaction to be gained in putting our values into action. Every time that you move eastwards, or every time you behave fairly, you are acting true to yourself and your values. The benefits to you of acting in accordance with your values are now.

g) Are personal, but often alike those of others

Any one person's values are likely to be similar to another's but will also differ in significant ways. Although there may be some general agreement about values in health and care work there it is likely that in situations where difficult decisions have to be made there will be some conflict about which value is to be prioritised. The classic example is the very common conflict between caring for people and allowing them to make their own possibly risky decisions.

There will very likely be a general agreement about personal values but each individual will hold and express them in their own particular way.

Personal values are also a bit different from professional values. Professional values are a non-negotiable part of our working lives. They reflect the very essence of our profession and are a very good guide to our professional conduct. However, unlike personal values, they come from other people, not from inside ourselves. They tend to be rather general and this can mean that they are sometimes a bit vague. They also are not arranged in any sense of priority.

Having said all that, most professionals will find that their personal values are in accord with their professional values. Sometimes they will have chosen that profession because it reflects their values and sometimes it will be because over the years they have taken in, or introjected, these professional values and made them part of their own self-concept.

h) Are complementary to professional values

For some of you, these values will be at the front of your mind and you will find it easy to describe and talk about them. Others will have their values residing in the back of your heads where they are less easy to put in to words, even if they are still effective there.

All of you will have personal values. It is these personal values that we are going to explore in this session.

Exercise 2.1: Writing my own retirement speech

Timing: 45 mins

Aim

Participants will reflect on their career, how it has been so far and how they wish it to be, from the point of view of the values they demonstrate in their work and how they would want to be regarded by their colleagues.

Materials

▶ Slide 2.13: My retirement speech

▶ Handout 2.1: Your own retirement speech

▶ A1 flipchart or whiteboard

▶ pens

Notes for the trainer

1. Show *Slide 2.13: My retirement speech*.

2. Distribute *Handout 2.1: Your own retirement speech*.

▶ Ask participants to imagine themselves in the future, at the point when they are in their final day at work prior to retirement. They are about to attend a small ceremony to mark this. A good friend and colleague of many years will be making a short speech. This is a time of goodwill towards you and gratitude for the service provided over the years.

▶ The task is for each participant to write down some bullet points of what, in their heart of hearts, they would really like to hear. What would a well-intentioned person who has known them over many years say about them as a person and as a professional? What is it about them that they would really like to be recognised and praised?

Allow 15 minutes for this part of the exercise.

3. Ask participants to get in to pairs with somebody they know and feel comfortable with and spend some time discussing what they have written down.

Allow 15 minutes for this part of the exercise.

4. Go round the room asking for contributions. Ask participants to give an example of a quality that they would like to be remembered for. Write each contribution down on the flipchart or whiteboard.

Allow 15 minutes for this part of the exercise.

Prompts and questions

Depending on the time available, ask some of the following questions:

▶ Was this a difficult task? Were there any surprises?

▶ Was there much difference in what each person in a pair wrote?

▶ Or similarities?

Points for the trainer to cover:

▶ None of these values are more right or wrong than any others.

▶ Although many of these values may be similar to professional values, they are not exactly the same.

Exercise 2.2: Choosing values from a list

Timing: 45 mins

Aim

▶ To select a number of values that they feel are personally most important to them

Materials

▶ Slide 2.14: Examples

▶ Handout 2.2: Choosing your own values

Notes for the trainer

1. Show *Slide 2.14: Examples*. Distribute copies of *Handout 2.2: Choosing your own values*.

2. Inform the participants that this exercise will complement the **Retirement speech** exercise that they have just done and also the **A good leader I have known** exercise (Session 1: Exercise 4) from the previous session. They will be shown a list of values. Bearing in mind what they have written from these previous two exercises, ask participants to indicate which values are most important to them at work.

▶ They should choose **no more than five** values as being Very Important to them, and should put a circle around these.

▶ They should then choose any values that are Moderately Important to them and should underline these.

▶ Remaining values that are not important and need not be marked.

If they can think of a value that is significant to them that is not listed here please ask them to write it in the final blank box at the bottom of Handout 2.2.

Allow 15 minutes for this part of the exercise.

3. Ask participants to get into pairs with a different person this time (but still someone they feel comfortable with) and spend some time discussing their choice of values.

Allow 15 minutes for this part of the exercise.

4. Bring the group back together again and discuss the exercise. Go round the room asking for contributions. Ask:

▶ Was it difficult choosing only five values?

▶ Was there much difference between their responses and their partner's?

▶ Were there any surprises?

▶ Is there much difference between the values they hold at work and the values they have outside of work?

Allow 15 minutes for this part of the exercise.

Prompts and questions

Depending on the time available, ask some of the following questions:

▶ Do you talk much about values at work?

▶ Do you assume that other people know what your values are? Do you know what theirs are?

▶ Are you beginning to see how values are important in determining performance in health?

Points for the trainer to cover

▶ The list of values are single words, they may be open to different interpretations by different people.

▶ None of these values are more right or wrong than any others.

▶ Although many of these values may be similar to professional values, they are not exactly the same.

Exercise 2.3: Realising values in my current work

Timing: 45 mins

Aim

▶ To consider the five most important values identified, and consider how they live these values in their current work

▶ To consider anything else that they can do to live these values a bit more

Materials

▶ Slide 2.15: Examples

▶ Handout 2.3a and b: Values in your daily work

Notes for the trainer

1. Distribute *Handout 2.3 (a and b): Values in your daily work.*

2. Explain that in the first part of this exercise participants will be asked to take the five most important values they have identified in the previous exercises and to reflect on how they put them into action – how they live these values in their day-to-day work.

3. Ask participants to complete the handout:

▶ In the first column of **Handout 2.3**, they should write their five chosen values.

▶ In the second column they should write what they do, any actions they take that show they are living this value, using this value as a guide, putting this value in to action.

It is important that the participants write down actions. Explain that what is required is things that people do or say. Actions or words that would be captured if they were being recorded on a video camera.

Thoughts, feelings and wishes are not required at this point.

4. Show *Slide 2.15: Examples.*

Explain that sitting with Mrs Smith and taking the Dementia Friends course are both actions. They could be seen by another person. This is how we know that somebody is living their values.

Allow 15 minutes for this part of the exercise.

5. Explain that the second part of the exercise is to write down one practical step participants could take to further show how they realise one of their values.

For this part of the exercise, ask the participants to get into pairs with somebody they feel at ease with. Ask them to choose two of these values and to make a plan for a concrete action that could be taken to make these values a little bit more evident in their working lives.

Emphasise that you are asking people to consider small changes. Nobody should be setting themselves a challenge that they cannot achieve with a little effort.

Allow 10 minutes for this part of the exercise.

6. Bring the group back together and ask each participant to read out the results of the discussion from the last exercise. That is, they should be encouraged to say,

    a. what value they are aiming to realise in their everyday work

    b. how they are planning to improve the way they live out that value at work by making a tiny step in the right direction.

Allow 20 minutes for this part of the exercise.

Prompts and questions

Depending on the time available, ask some of the following questions:

▶ How well does their chosen value guide their choice of action?

▶ Although acting in a way that is consistent with one's values leads to a sense of satisfaction, do they foresee any difficulties, any discomfort?

Points for the trainer to cover

▶ Make sure they talk about actions, things they will do or say.

▶ Encourage plans be made for small steps only.

Session summary

Timing: 15 mins

Aim

▶ To summarise and remind participants of the session's content and their contributions

▶ To point out how the material produced by them illustrates the importance of values in care work and this in turn fits in with the whole Good Care Leadership course

Materials

▶ Slide 2.16: Personal Values: Parts of leadership

▶ Slide 2.17: Personal Values: The nature of values

▶ Slide 2.18: Personal Values: Retirement speech

▶ Slide 2.19: Personal Values: List of values

▶ Slide 2.20: Personal Values: Values in action

▶ Slide 2.21: Personal values (III)

Notes for the trainer

1. Show *Slide 2.16: Personal Values: Parts of leadership*.

Tell the group that it is now time for a summary of the session.

The first point to remember is that values are an important part of being a leader for great care at the clinical frontline. Along with the other three components (Confidence and competence, Authority, and Motivating others) knowing your values and being able to live them out in your work is essential for the provision of great care.

Everybody in this room will have a set of personal values that are suited to health and care work. This session has aimed to give you an opportunity to discuss and reflect on your values and the part they play in your working life.

2. Show *Slide 2.17: Personal Values: The nature of values*.

▶ Remind the participants that we discussed the nature of values and the way they give meaning to work; also, that values are not 'goals'. Values may never be fully achieved/realised; they are only lived out day after day. Values are always in action. More of a direction of travel rather than a destination.

▶ Remind participants that the values we have been talking about are personal values. These are often similar to professional values (which we must remember are not optional). Often, professional values are fully adopted or incorporated into your own personality. Saying, *"I care. That's just what I do"* may be expressing a value the person has held from childhood, or it may be a value they have come to absorb over years as a professional or it may be a bit of both.

▶ Personal values tend to be a bit more idiosyncratic, more tied to strong emotions and personal motivation.

3. Show *Slide 2.18: Personal Values: Retirement speech*.

▶ We looked at the personal nature of values by seeing what people would like to hear about themselves at their retirement speech. Much more than achievements, it is usually the values that drive you that others will remember and cherish.

4. Show *Slide 2.19: Personal Values: List of values*.

Remind the group how we also looked over a list of values and considered which were the five most important values to them. Inevitably, this involved some prioritising and leaving some values off the list. The purpose of this is to make it clear that each person holds some values dearer than others. This is a point to bear in mind as it may lead to conflict, within yourself or between yourself and others.

5. Show *Slide 2.20: Personal Values: Values in action*.

▶ Values are significant when they are put into action. Remind participants of the exercise looking at the ways in which a person's values are often put in to action through hundreds of different acts over a working day. Most of these will be small acts, but if they are driven by a strong moral value, they will never be insignificant. We then looked at how each participant could do something small to show that they were realising two chosen values in their work.

▶ Ask participants to take care of the notes they made here as they may come in useful in Session 5.

6. Show *Slide 2.21: Personal values*.

Good quality care is provided where staff meet patients or residents. It is what the staff do and the way they do it that determines the quality of care delivered. A strong sense of values that are lived out and put in to action is a great guide to excellent care. Values are something that all members of staff already have. This session has only been a reminder and a time for reflection.

Thank the group for their participation and their contributions. Ask if there are any questions.

Session 3: Use of Authority

Timing: 3 hours

Overview

Participants are introduced to the idea that interpersonal authority, power and influence stem from many sources, only one of which may be the rank or position held within an organisation. Even staff low in the hierarchy can stand up for good quality care.

For some, the exercise of authority will be easy and natural. Others may find that doing so moves them out of their 'comfort zone'.

Activity	Time required
Introduction to the session	10 mins
Introduction to the necessity of using your authority	10 mins
Introduction to the five types of power	25 mins
Exercise 3.1: Case study	30 mins
Exercise 3.2: Using power appropriately	45 mins
Exercise 3.3: Feeling comfortable with each of these types of power	40 mins
The special moral responsibilities of leaders	10 mins
Session summary	10 mins

Materials

▶ Slides 3.1 to 3.25

▶ Handouts 3.1 to 3.11

▶ A1 flipchart

▶ pens

Introduction to the session

Timing: 10 mins

Aims

▶ To welcome the participants to the training

▶ To inform them of the programme for the session

▶ To make personal introductions

Materials

▶ Slides 3.1 to 3.3

▶ A1 flipchart

▶ pens

Notes for the trainer

1. Show *Slide 3.1: Welcome*.

▶ Welcome learners back to the session, introducing yourself and giving participants some background information about yourself as appropriate.

▶ Outline housekeeping arrangements, such as the procedure in the event of a fire, the mobile phone policy and the location of toilets etc.

2. Show and read out *Slide 3.2: Programme*. Tell participants that there is a lot to fit in so you will need to keep to the timings listed, but that within these constraints you will welcome questions at any point in the proceedings.

3. Show *Slide 3.3: Four components of good care leadership*. Explain that this is the third of four sessions in this training looking at a different one of the four components of good care leadership. All four sessions interact and overlap and all are necessary.

Introduction to the necessity of using your authority

Timing: 10 mins

Aims

▶ To familiarise participants with the idea that the exercise of power and influence is inevitable in work situations (indeed in most social situations)

▶ To explain that one of the ways they have of influencing workplace culture is through the use of their personal power or authority, however strong or mild this might be

Materials

▶ Slide 3.4: Ward culture

▶ Slide 3.5: Culture change

▶ Slide 3.6: The power of the individual

Notes for the trainer

1. Show *Slide 3.4: Ward culture*.

Explain that in every workplace, whether this is a ward, a clinic or a care home, there is a culture that is in large part created by the people who work there. These are not the only contributors to the workplace culture. Other factors include policies, professional guidelines, funding, staffing levels and workload. Everybody in that workplace will be affected by that culture. Equally, everybody in that workplace has the potential to mould that culture.

The important questions are:

▶ Will that influence be weak or strong?

▶ Will that influence be for good or for ill?

Usually, the higher-ranking staff will have the strongest influence, but this is far from inevitable.

2. Show *Slide 3.5: Culture change*

▶ Cultures can (sometimes) change quickly. Explain that the quote on the slide is taken from an account of a ward where there was poor quality care, a lack of respect and little kindness for older people. Yet the presence of just one nurse made all the difference.

The 'culture' of this ward was not great, far from person-centred. Yet it all changed with one person.

▶ Ask the participants if, *without giving names*, they know of any wards/clinics/care homes they would be happy to be admitted into, and any that they would rather avoid? Use their answers as an indication that cultures can vary from ward to ward within a Trust or from care home to care home.

▶ Ask participants if, *without giving names*, they know of a ward/clinic/care home where they are happier if one particular nurse is on duty rather than another? Use their answers as an indication that cultures can vary from ward to ward, day to day, shift to shift, even in the same workplace.

3. Show **Slide 3.6: The power of the individual**.

▶ Explain that this shows what happened when a volunteer in an experiment was sitting with another person (a confederate of the experimenter) filling in forms when a loud crash and cries of distress came from next door. The response of the volunteer depended hugely on what the confederate said. When the confederate said *"I don't think this has anything to do with us. Perhaps it is another experiment,"* only a quarter of the volunteers attempted to go next door to offer help. In contrast, when the confederate said *"This sounds bad. I'll go and find the person in charge; you go in and see what happened"* then every single one went to offer help.

▶ The point to be made is that people look to others to understand what is going on in uncertain situations. Everyone here has influence and can help turn other people from passive bystanders into active helpers, depending on how they react.

▶ So, we can see that all of us have the power to influence others to some degree. We can influence individuals and we can influence a workgroup culture. It is inevitable. The important questions are whether your influence will be strong or weak and whether it will be for good or for ill?

▶ Some people find it easy to use their authority and influence. Others are a bit more reluctant to do so. Ask participants to consider the work they have done on Confidence and Competence, and on Personal Values (Sessions 1 and 2) to help them here. Often wielding authority and power is uncomfortable, but confidence in what you are doing and knowing it is guided by clear values will be an invaluable help.

▶ Say that using your authority does not simply mean shouting at people and telling them what to do. To illustrate this, we shall look at the ways that power or authority can be used at work.

Introduction to the five types of power

Timing: 25 mins

Aims

▶ To introduce the classification of the five types of power at work

▶ To show some ways in which each type of power may be used

Materials

▶ Slide 3.7: Legitimate/positional power

▶ Slide 3.8: Using legitimate/positional power

▶ Slide 3.9: Reward power

▶ Slide 3.10: Using reward power

▶ Slide 3.11: Coercive power

▶ Slide 3.12: Using coercive power

▶ Slide 3.13: Expert power

▶ Slide 3.14: Using expert power

▶ Slide 3.15: Referent power

▶ Slide 3.16: Using referent power

Notes for the trainer

1. Show the slides with the following commentary

Legitimate or positional power

1. Show *Slide 3.7: Legitimate/positional power*.

▶ This is the power that comes with the holding of a position of formal authority. It is usually explicitly stated in official documents and is also accepted as a norm within the organisation. Legitimate power can be backed up with organisational sanctions like disciplinary procedures. Usually, things do not go that far because of its widespread acceptance. The extent of a person's positional power is usually defined in organisational documents, such as job descriptions. It is usually clear from a person's rank or title.

▶ Legitimate power can be challenged directly if requests contradict the basic principles (values) of the organisation or larger society.

▶ It may also be challenged indirectly by delay or evasion in carrying out the task. If this is successful, further disobedience is likely.

▶ Junior staff usually expect somebody senior to them to take the lead. However, this power needs to be wielded thoughtfully as, on the one hand, heavy handedness can breed resentment while, on the other, being hesitant can be seen as weakness.

2. Show *Slide 3.8: Using legitimate/positional power*.

As a general rule, legitimate power is best used when:

▶ You are polite and respectful towards juniors and requests are made in a way that does not cause resentment.

▶ The reasons for requests and orders are explained and not made in an arbitrary manner.

▶ The request or order is clear. You make sure the person you are instructing understands fully. If lengthy or complicated, requests or orders may be written down.

▶ The request is within the scope of your authority and, if necessary, you can verify the legitimacy of the request.

▶ Proper channels are followed as set out in your organisation.

▶ The request is followed up and compliance verified. Sometimes people hesitate before carrying out unpleasant tasks and it will be necessary to follow up on your request to ensure compliance.

Reward power

3. Show *Slide 3.9: Reward power*.

▶ This is the power to control valuable rewards. Most healthcare leaders do not have the power to offer monetary or similar rewards to their staff. They may be able to wield power over such things as references, access to training, better work schedules and so on.

▶ Above all, leaders, and indeed all of us, have the power at our disposal to reward other people socially through our attention and approval. Indeed, so long as this form of influence is used genuinely, it is very powerful. Not because people need your approval (some do, some do not) but because they like to be noticed. It is the best way of letting people know that you are paying attention to what they are doing and what they are doing is correct.

4. Show *Slide 3.10: Using reward power*.

As a general rule, reward power is best used when:

▶ You are guided by fairness and avoid any favouritism.

▶ You do not promise more than you can give.

▶ Rewards are tied clearly to specific actions.

▶ The reward is valued by the person (don't buy the team doughnuts if most of them are on a diet).

▶ It is delivered in an appropriate way. Wild enthusiastic praise may be suitable for a first-year trainee, a silent nod may be sufficient for a more senior person.

▶ You make a point of noticing good work.

▶ You praise far more often than criticise. A ratio of four positive remarks to one criticism is fine.

▶ You are genuine in any praise you give. This is not a way of manipulating people, it is simply the right and respectful way to treat people doing a difficult (and often thankless) job.

Coercive power

5. Show *Slide 3.11: Coercive power*.

▶ Explain that this is the power to inflict some sort of punishment or pressure. At its most formal it involves the exercise of power through the organisation's disciplinary procedures.

▶ But if we understand that a punishment may mean *anything* that is unpleasant to an individual, we can see that many types of less formal coercion are commonplace, from a frown to a full dressing down.

▶ Just like social rewards, social disapproval can take many forms and needs to be appropriate.

▶ Before using any form of coercive power it is important to know that the team are absolutely clear about what is expected of them.

▶ The use of coercive power tends to result in mere compliance rather than wholehearted commitment. It may also result in resentment and resistance.

6. Show *Slide 3.12: Using coercive power*.

As a general rule coercive power is most effective when:

▶ Standards are clear and known to everybody. Although ignorance of the rules is no excuse, it is important that everybody is clear about what is expected. This is important when 'unwritten rules' have become established.

▶ Lapses from standards are responded to quickly and not tolerated. If people are not corrected for failures they may come to believe that you approve of their actions. Or worse, that you don't care.

▶ The behaviour is criticised, not the person. Personal attacks (eg "You are lazy") provoke anger and are easily contradicted by counter examples. Be specific about what you think somebody did wrong.

▶ Try not to criticise in public. Humiliating people creates resentment and resistance. Whilst it is important to let others know that you are dealing with an infraction, it is not necessary to make a display.

▶ Accompany your criticism with suggestions to help the person improve. Criticism only lets people know what not to do. It is helpful to show them what is needed and, if necessary, make it easier for them to do the right thing.

▶ Warnings are followed up on. If you do need to add a warning about future conduct, it is important that this is credible and acted upon. Empty threats only diminish your authority.

Expert power

7. Show *Slide 3.13: Expert power*

Having a special expertise can confer power, especially if that expertise is rare, valued and relevant in the work situation. People who know the best way to perform a procedure and who are up to date with professional developments will have more expert power than those who do not. It may be necessary to show that your expertise is both important and not easily available from other sources.

A crucial aspect of expert power is that it is limited to your area of expertise. Knowing much about, for example, diabetes care, may allow you to take a lead with diabetic patients, but it does not confer any such power in any other area. Similarly, if you wish to remain credible it is essential that you acknowledge limits to your expertise, you do not exceed yourself and you do not bluff.

8. Show *Slide 3.14 Using expert power*.

▶ Unless you are widely recognised as an expert in your field you many need to demonstrate your expertise by providing information and evidence to support your suggestions. You may also need to show your qualifications. Describing previous examples of success can also be helpful.

▶ As an 'expert' you must know what you are talking about. It is important you stay up to date with your subject area.

▶ Requests, proposals or orders should be given confidently. There is little hesitation or havering. Do not make contradictory or inconsistent statements.

▶ You do not lecture or harangue. Explaining something, especially something you are enthusiastic about, may lead to a long speech that may imply that you think the other person is ignorant.

▶ You acknowledge that, whatever your field of expertise, other people will have some knowledge, some skills and certainly some opinions.

▶ You admit the limits of your expertise. You do not know everything even within your chosen field. Saying "I don't know" is nothing to be ashamed of.

Referent power

9. Show *Slide 3.15: Referent power*.

▶ This stems from other people's desire to please or emulate a person who they admire and respect. Often this is due to their high professional and clinical standards, but it can also be personal and idiosyncratic. The person with referent power is felt to be 'on our side'. Everybody can aim to stimulate some respect and loyalty from members of their team.

▶ The strongest form of referent power is when others try to emulate a role model and will consequently respond positively to their suggestions, and will try to be like that person in behaviour and in attitudes. In many cases, followers of a person with referent power will anticipate requests and spontaneously attempt to behave in the way that person would wish.

▶ You may feel this does not apply to you, that your team takes very little notice of what you say and the example you set. Nonetheless, it is likely that they will be watching everything you do and judging everything you say.

▶ An important aspect of referent power is that it tends to elicit full commitment from other team members. That is other people personally identify with the behaviour, attitudes and values of the person holding referent power. More than any other type of power it does not simply elicit mere compliance.

10. Show *Slide 3.16 Using referent power*.

▶ Referent power is gained and held by showing concern for the rest of the team, showing trust and dealing fairly with them.

▶ It also depends upon your integrity which is demonstrated by behaving in a way that is consistent with your declared values.

▶ Being a consistent role model is important if you wish to use referent power (but you must also be aware that people will imitate less desirable behaviour shown by someone they respect).

▶ Actions speak louder than words and you will be judged not so much on what you say but far more on what you do. This takes time.

Exercise 3.1: Case study

Timing: 30 mins

Aims

▶ To illustrate one way that the theoretical concepts of 'sources of power' are put into action

▶ To encourage the group to discuss the ways that the five types of power are used

Materials

▶ Handout 3.1: A clinical case study

Notes for the trainer

1. Give out *Handout 3.1: A clinical case study*.

▶ Explain that, in Handout 3.1, there is the answer given by a senior hospital nurse in response to the question "How do you ensure your teams give good care?" This woman was in charge of over one hundred nurses working in a hospital unit and four bases in the community.

▶ Request that, as they read this account, they mark any examples of:

   1. legitimate power

   2. reward power

   3. coercive power

   4. expert power

   5. referent power.

This could be done by underlining phrases and putting initials like LP or RewP in the margin.

▶ Explain that some of what she says may reflect the use of more than one source of power.

Allow 10 minutes for this part of the exercise.

2. After 10 minutes call the group together again and ask them for any examples that they have found of the five types of power.

Use the following as a reference:

TYPE OF POWER	EXAMPLE
Legitimate/ positional power Sharing Legitimate Power (LP) Using LP autocratically (with reluctance) Using LP with her own managers	I take my responsibility for the service very seriously. I do try to share decision making. We have had quite a few ballots on issues, where all staff have got to 'vote' on a matter. Other decisions are thrashed out at meetings. Occasionally, I think there are decisions that just have to be made and I'm happy to do that. Part of a manager's job is to protect staff from stress. For me this is about fighting battles with the next layer up.
Reward power Much evidence of social rewards, verbal and written Also her thoughts on being genuine and not manipulative	I, and the managers who work under me, all try to give positive verbal and written feedback to staff for good work done… …and to mention it in staff meetings… …and the monthly newsletter positive about them, respectful towards them, I believe that giving praise to people for working hard and doing well **is the right thing to do**. It's not a management ploy, or a 'tactic' to get people to work harder. Neither is it about trying to be popular. It's about human being to human being respect and valuing colleagues as whole people who bring their whole selves to their jobs and give of themselves every day. My belief is, and I might be horribly deluded, that staff here appreciate being praised and thanked. they praise and thank others (I hear it happening all the time, not directed by me)
Coercive power Prepared to enforce standards	I then tear them off a strip in private
Expert power Displaying high level of professional credibility	I do shifts, on calls, come in in the middle of the night, go to home visits. As someone said to me recently, 'we know you would never ask us to do anything that you would not do yourself.'

Referent power	I am rostered for 1 shift per week only, but I am counted in the numbers for the shift so I'm not supernumerary.
Being someone the team can look up to, can trust and respect. Keeping them safe. Being on their side	when they get a letter from me they can trust it, because they see me in action every day and, most of the time, I act in the same way. That is, positive about them, respectful towards them, never slagging anyone off to them and never slagging them off to anyone else
	I guess part of them trusting me is that I am out there with them
	I do try to share decision making. We have had quite a few ballots on issues, where all staff have got to 'vote' on a matter. Other decisions are thrashed out at meetings
	… part of a manager's job is to protect staff from stress

3. Ask the group to give examples of sources of power that they have identified. Ask in turn for examples of:

▶ legitimate power

▶ reward power

▶ coercive power

▶ expert power

▶ referent power.

Ask what the group think of the frequency with which each type of power is mentioned? For example, the single mention of 'coercive power' and the many mentions of 'reward power'.

Prompts and questions

Depending on the time available ask some of the following questions:

▶ Can they think of ways they could use any of these practices in their own work?

▶ What value is there in having facility with several types of power in your toolkit?

Points for the trainer

▶ The service this woman ran was considered one of the best in the country.

▶ Her 'expert power', as described by her, was no more than being competent in her field.

▶ Her answer covers only part of what leaders do. It is likely that in a short reply she wrote about what she considered to be the most important aspects of leading.

Exercise 3.2: Using power appropriately

Timing: 45 mins

Aim

▶ Participants will consider the ways that various types of power, authority and influence may be used in their day-to-day work. This will involve both examples of the ways that such power is actually used and to suggest ways that it might be used.

Materials

Part 1

▶ Handout 3.2: Legitimate or positional power

▶ Handout 3.3: Reward power

▶ Handout 3.4: Coercive power

▶ Handout 3.5: Expert power

▶ Handout 3.6: Referent power

Part 2

▶ Handout 3.7: Using legitimate/positional power

▶ Handout 3.8: Using reward power

▶ Handout 3.9: Using coercive power

▶ Handout 3.10: Using expert power

▶ Handout 3.11: Using referent power

▶ flipchart or whiteboard, A1 paper

▶ pens

Notes for the trainer

Part 1

1. Split the participants in to five roughly equal groups.

Explain that this activity is for each group to explore how one of the five types of power are used in their everyday work.

2. Give out a sheet of flipchart or A1 paper and some pens to each group.

3. Allocate each group a 'type of power' to work on.

▶ For the group allocated 'Legitimate power' hand out copies of *Handout 3.2: Legitimate or positional power*

▶ For the group allocated 'Reward power' hand out copies of *Handout 3.3: Reward power*

▶ For the group allocated 'Coercive power' hand out copies of *Handout 3.4: Coercive power*

▶ For the group allocated 'Expert power' hand out copies of *Handout 3.5: Expert power*

▶ For the group allocated 'Referent power' hand out copies of *Handout 3.6: Referent power*

Ask for one member of each group to write down the ideas that the group comes with.

4. Explain you would like each group to come up with examples of how the type of power that they have been allocated is used in work situations. For this they can draw on their own personal experience of how they use this power and also how other people use power (including the case study above).

They may also consider some good ways that each type of power could be used even if they have not seen this use in practice.

5. For example, the 'legitimate power' group might suggest witnessing a Matron insisting a hoist is used when the HCA was in a rush and wanted to do without. The 'expert power' group might give the example of how a Speech and Language Therapist implemented a new way of reminding people with swallowing difficulties to take a sip of water with each mouthful of food, even though she had no formal power within the care home.

Allow 20 minutes for this part of the exercise.

Part 2

1. Call the larger group back together again.

2. Distribute *Handouts 3.7–3.11* to each participant.

▶ Explain that these handouts contain some brief notes in the left-hand column showing some good ways of implementing the particular source of power or authority and we will be using them for a self-assessment exercise shortly. There are also some blank rows at the bottom and these are spaces for ideas generated by the small groups.

▶ Ask for feedback from the small groups in turn, asking them for examples that they have generated for ways that the different types of power can be used. Some of these group-generated ideas will overlap with the ideas on the handouts; some will be novel. Discuss these and encourage participants to write down ideas from this discussion on to the relevant handout.

Allow 25 minutes for this exercise.

Prompts and questions

Depending on the time available ask some of the following questions:

▶ Have there ever been unexpected or unwanted consequences when using this type of power?

▶ How do others use their power over you? How does this make you feel?

▶ If you feel someone is using their power inappropriately, can you think of any ways to regain your sense of control?

▶ Are you ever wholly powerless?

Points for the trainer

▶ The use of power in all its forms is inevitable in working life. The abuse of power is not.

▶ Some forms of power are more appropriate to some circumstances.

▶ Being confident makes the exercise of power more comfortable.

▶ The use of coercive power is best kept to a minimum, but it remains an essential part of leadership when poor care is witnessed.

Exercise 3.3: Feeling comfortable with each of these types of power

1. Each participant now has five handouts (Handouts 3.7– 3.11) with some ideas culled from the larger group entered on each sheet.

▶ The first part of this exercise is entirely personal. Ask participants to go through the five handouts to score themselves on each of the various ways of using power, as indicated in the far-left column on each handout sheet. For each way of using power they should score themselves as using it 'Mostly' or 'Sometimes' or 'Rarely' and also indicate whether they are comfortable using this method with a Y or a N in the final column.

▶ Any items that do not apply should be left blank.

Allow 15 minutes for this part of the exercise.

2. Ask each participant to choose two 'Ways of using power'. One that they feel fully comfortable using and one that they feel very uncomfortable using. Ask them to get in to pairs and discuss with their partner:

▶ Any differences that they notice between the two 'Ways of using power' they have chosen.

▶ Whether they tend to over rely on ways they are comfortable with or avoid ways they are not comfortable with, or both.

▶ Any changes they might wish to make.

Allow 10 minutes for this exercise.

3. Call the larger group back together again.

Ask for any comments on this exercise.

Prompts and questions

Depending on the time available ask some of the following questions:

▶ How many people feel comfortable or uncomfortable with forms of legitimate, reward, coercive, expert and referent power?

▶ Does anybody feel comfortable with all of these types of power?

▶ Does anybody feel uncomfortable with all of these types of power?

Points for the trainer

▶ Concern about not being liked is common. This concern should be put in perspective by considering what may happen to standards of care if the use of power is shunned.

▶ Discomfort is common in some use of power. This is inevitable if you leave your comfort zone. Leaving your comfort zone is necessary if you are to change and grow.

▶ Followers expect leaders to use their power and will be disappointed if you do not.

Allow 15 minutes for this part of the exercise.

The special moral responsibilities of leaders

Say that with power comes responsibility. Although everybody can potentially do some good or cause some harm to the people in their care, this potential is increased enormously the more power you have as a leader. When you influence other people your power for good or for ill is enormously increased.

For example, Harold Shipman, possibly the most prolific mass murderer ever, killed as many as 250 people, operating on his own over 21 years. Whereas an under-performing Trust board at Mid-Staffordshire NHS Foundation Trust were responsible for between 400 and 1200 excess patient deaths in just three years.

There are some special moral challenges that come with the exercise of power that need to be considered.

1. Show *Slide 3.17: Moral challenges*.

    1. The temptation to use one's power for personal gain. There are a few opportunities for material gain open to leaders in healthcare and these opportunities increase with increasing power. More common are opportunities for either an easy life or for self-promotion.

    2. **The temptation to harm others**. Power allows a person more opportunities to cause hurt or harm to people they are ill-intentioned towards. This hostility may be caused by personal prejudice, it may be provoked by the other person's behaviour or it may be that other people get in the way of our goals and plans. Also, sadly, some people are bullies. This is a serious challenge to moral leadership and needs to be checked by compassion and tolerance.

    3. **The avoidance of injustice**. To use power of any sort is to risk using it inequitably. People in your team will care a lot about fairness and will be very sensitive to deviations from it. Unfairness results in low morale, lowered motivation and possibly resentment. To avoid an unfair use of power one must constantly pay attention to the effects of one's decisions and judgments, even of one's non-decisions.

    4. **The need to rise to the challenge**. Leaders need to use their powers not just to keep their work unit running smoothly but also to respond effectively to any unforeseen events or problems that emerge. Leadership is creative and adaptive. This will be a challenge as the priorities of running a ward or a home may clash with the special needs of the specific situation that occurs.

Session summary

Timing: 10 mins

Aim

▶ To summarise and remind participants of the session's content and their contributions

▶ To point out how the material produced by them fits with the concept of the appropriate use of authority to influence the work culture for the better

▶ To show how this fits in with the whole Good Care Leadership course

Materials

▶ Slides 3.18 to 3.25

Notes for the trainer

1. Say that this is a quick reminder of the contents of the session and how all parts relate to each other.

2. Show **Slide 3.18 to 3.25: Use of authority**, one slide at a time.

Slide 3.18: The first point to remember is that using your authority is an important part of being a leader for great care at the clinical frontline. Along with the other three components (Confidence and competence, Values and Motivating others) being comfortable in the appropriate use of authority is essential for the provision of great care.

Slide 3.19: Say how every individual on a ward or in a care home contributes to the 'culture'. There are external influences too, but much of the culture is made by the people present. This can vary from ward to ward, care home to care home. It can also vary from day to day depending on who is on duty. Every member of staff influences the culture. The important questions are 'Will your influence be weak or strong?' and 'Will your influence be for the better or for the worse?'

Slide 3.20: Say how you may feel powerless, especially the junior staff. Yet it is clear that in some circumstances it is possible to shake people out of being passive, uncaring bystanders just by what you say.

Slide 3.21: Refer to your introduction on the five types of power at work and remind participants that you have discussed them at some length. Some types of power come with your rank or position. Legitimate power comes with your position. Reward power and coercive power are to do with rewards and punishments. We talked a lot about verbal rewards and reprimands. Expert power comes with your knowledge and experience. It is not so much a matter of being 'The World Expert' but more about being professional and competent and knowing what you are doing. Finally, referent power is when your good example inspires others to want to follow your lead.

Informal rewards, expert power and referent power are generally best for motivating others. When you need to gain compliance, coercive power is effective but may lead to resentment and resistance so should be used carefully.

Slide 3.22: Remind the group of the case study of the senior nurse and how they discussed her use of the five types of power – which ones she used most, which she barely mentioned.

Slide 3.23: Remind participants that you have looked at examples of how power is used in everyday working life. Some examples appeared to be more helpful and effective than others.

Slide 3.24: We considered how comfortable each of us is with the different types of power. How sometimes it is difficult to use one or other of them and this involves moving out of our comfort zones. Yet research shows that leaders who are able to use all five are more effective.

Slide 3.25: We considered the moral challenges inherent in being a leader, in the use of power and the ability to influence other people. By doing so, our potential for causing harm is greatly increased and we must be careful how we use power, whatever type it is. These are just four of the most important ways that people who are careless in the use of their power have gone astray.

Thank the group for their participation and their contributions. Ask if there are any questions.

Session 4: Motivating Others

Timing: 2 hours 45 minutes

Overview

This session will approach the essential leadership task of encouraging motivation in the participants' junior colleagues and peer group. It will build on the three previous sessions **Confidence and Competence**, **Values** and **Using Power Appropriately** as well as introducing the new concept of **Belongingness**.

Participants will be asked to reflect that all they have learned in the previous sessions as relevant to improving their own performance will also be relevant to members of their teams.

Activity	Time required
Introduction to the session	10 mins
Introduction to junk and wholesome motivation	20 mins
Exercise 4.1: Supporting confidence and competence	40 mins
Exercise 4.2: Supporting values and meaning	40 mins
Exercise 4.3: Supporting 'belongingness'	40 mins
Session summary	15 mins

Materials

▶ Slides 4.1–4.19

▶ Handouts 4.1–4.4

▶ A1 flipchart

▶ pens

Introduction to the session

Timing: 10 mins

Aims

▶ To welcome the participants to the training

▶ To inform them of the programme for this session

▶ To put the session's training in the context of the larger programme

Materials

▶ Slide 4.1: Welcome

▶ Slide 4.2: Programme

▶ Slide 4.3: Four components of good care leadership

Notes for the trainer

1. Show *Slide 4.1: Welcome*.

▶ Welcome learners to the training session, introducing yourself and giving participants some background information about yourself, as appropriate.

▶ Outline housekeeping arrangements, such as the procedure in the event of a fire, the mobile phone policy and the location of toilets etc.

2. Show and read out *Slide 4.2: Programme* and inform participants that there is a lot to fit in so you will need to keep to the timings listed, but that within these constraints you will welcome questions at any point in the proceedings.

3. Show *Slide 4.3: Four components of good care leadership*. Explain that this session is the last of four sessions in this training looking at a different one of the four components of good care leadership. All four sessions interact and overlap and all are necessary.

4. Explain that the material covered in the first three sessions will be highly relevant to this session. These earlier sessions were designed to help build on your motivation for good care. You will be able to take what you have learned in these sessions and use it in your dealings with colleagues and juniors to build on their motivation.

Introduction to junk and wholesome motivation

Timing: 20 mins

Aims

▶ To explain that what the participants have learned about improving their own performance in the last three sessions will be equally applicable to their junior staff and colleagues; to motivate others they can apply the lessons of the past three sessions in their dealings with others

▶ To make the distinction between two types of motivation and to encourage participants to support and build inner motivation among their teams

▶ To discuss the matter of unmotivated staff

Materials

▶ Slide 4.4: Complete lack of motivation

▶ Slide 4.5: Junk food motivation (1)

▶ Slide 4.6: Junk food motivation (2)

▶ Slide 4.7: Wholesome motivation (1)

▶ Slide 4.8: Wholesome motivation (2)

Notes for the trainer

1. Explain that in the last three sessions we have been exploring Confidence and Competence, Personal Values and Use of Authority in the quest to make you the best frontline leader that you can be. In other words, these sessions have been about individual development.

▶ This session is about using your leadership skills to get the very best from your team, that is, it is about team development. There is a considerable overlap between the material in this session and that from the previous sessions. After all, what brings out the best in you is likely to bring out the best in the rest of your team, with some tweaking for individual strengths and needs naturally.

▶ Motivation comes in varying forms as well as in varying strengths. To simplify matters today we are going to talk about two general types of motivation, 'Junk Food' motivation and 'Wholesome' motivation. Like junk food and wholesome food they both provide energy and nutrition, but over time wholesome food is better for you and has fewer untoward effects.

But first we need to acknowledge that there are sometimes people at work who show no sign of being motivated at all – these people say things such as those listed in the next slide.

2. Show **Slide 4.4: Complete lack of motivation**.

▶ Ask the group if they can think of reasons why people might be this way and say such things. Encourage discussion with prompts such as:

   ▶ They are reacting to a poor work environment

   ▶ They are reacting to poor leadership

   ▶ They are excluded from the rest of the team

   ▶ Nobody has explained to them the importance of the job they are doing

   ▶ They are depressed and need help

   ▶ Finally, they are simply in the wrong job

▶ If you do have such unmotivated people in your team then you do definitely have a problem. However, it is worth considering that in some cases the cause will lie in the work situation (broadly defined), and sometimes in the person themselves. Either way, it may be possible to do something for them.

3. Show **Slide 4.5: Junk food motivation (1)**. The first type of junk food motivation comes from the excessive use of rewards and punishments by management, sometimes known as 'carrots and sticks'. These sorts of motivational strategies are very popular, yet when people are being employed to do work with any need for thought, judgement, expertise and interpersonal skills, these strategies have consistently been shown to be ineffective. Carrots and sticks are great for increasing performance on simple, repetitive, mechanical tasks. For higher level tasks, like giving care to complex patients in a busy environment, rewards and punishments are of little use.

▶ There are two unintended consequences of a carrot and stick approach. The first is demotivation, where somewhat paradoxically, people find that their natural motivation for a task or job is actually reduced if they feel they are being manipulated into doing it or that they are under the control of someone who is rewarding them for doing it. The second is 'gaming', in which they only put effort in to those parts of the job that their managers reward or punish, while other, maybe equally important, parts of the job are neglected.

▶ Comment on the phrases that people under 'Carrots and stick' motivation use – these are at the bottom of the slide. Ask participants if they recognise these.

4. Show **Slide 4.6: Junk food motivation (2)**. The second type of junk food motivation is the 'Inner critic'. Many people have an inner critic, but some people have a very powerful one. Whilst it is definitely a source of motivation, it is often associated with worry, discomfort and feelings of shame.

▶ If intense enough, the inner critic can lead people to be rigid, to avoid difficult situations due to a fear of failure and to develop a general sense of anxiety and insecurity.

▶ Comment on the phrases that people under Inner Critic motivation use, these are at the bottom of the slide. Ask participants if they recognise these.

▶ Remind participants that these are definitely types of motivation. They are very common and not to be rejected out of hand. However, they can be improved upon.

5. Show *Slide 4.7: Wholesome motivation (1)*.

This type of motivation is associated with high and persistent energy at work and with feelings of well-being among staff. It is the sort of motivation that springs from within. We see a lot of this in the healthcare systems, people who come to work week after week to do a difficult job because of their commitment to high standards of care.

▶ Wholesome motivation comes from within and reflects either a person's inner values and sense of identity or a sense of excitement and interest in the job. Since few jobs are exciting or interesting all the time a sense of the value of the job will help get people through the boring or unpleasant times.

▶ It is clearly preferable to have a team that shows Wholesome motivation most of the time

6. Show *Slide 4.8: Wholesome motivation (2)*.

Point out that, as wholesome motivation comes from within an individual, it cannot be forced. Fortunately, in healthcare, the great majority of people already have a strong inner drive to do a great job at caring one way or another. This drive may have been supressed, neglected or forgotten over the years, but it will be there in some form. The task of clinical frontline leaders is to nurture this inner wholesome motivation in their teams. In the following exercises we will be exploring some ways you can do this.

Exercise 4.1: Supporting confidence and competence

Timing: 40 mins

Aims

▶ To remind participants of the Session 1 exercises for enhancing confidence and competence

▶ To brainstorm other ways that confidence and competence can be nurtured in others in everyday work

Materials

▶ Slide 4.9: Three components of wholesome motivation (1)

▶ Slide 4.10: Confidence and competence

▶ Slide 4.11: Supporting confidence and competence

▶ Handout 4.1: Supporting confidence and competence

▶ 3 X A1 sheets of paper / a flipchart

▶ marker pens

Notes for the trainer

We have seen from the earlier sessions that one of the components of clinical leadership is a sense of confidence and competence at work. We have every reason to believe that if we wish others to show the same degree of enthusiasm and motivation at work that they will need a similar sense of confidence and competence.

1. Show *Slide 4.9: Three components of wholesome motivation (1)*.

▶ Explain that the exercises that were done in Session 1: Confidence and Competence might be used by leaders at work. Yet they were classroom exercises and do require time and preparation. There are many other ways of helping to build a sense of confidence and competence in your team. Many of you will practising some of these already.

▶ Explain that this is a brainstorming exercise. Use all that you know from your experience and all that you have learned from the past sessions, especially but not only Session 1. The task is for you to come up with some practical ways of supporting the confidence and competence of your frontline team. That is, things they can say and things they can do.

2. Show *Slide 4.10: Confidence and competence* which will be a reminder of the exercises in Session 1. As appropriate, say a few words to remind the participants that:

▶ We looked at the many achievements they have to their credit

▶ We considered three challenges that they have dealt with, or are maybe still dealing with

▶ We then thought about a good leader they have known and what they have learned from this person

Everyone in the group ranked themselves from zero to ten on a scale of how good they are and then spent time saying why they gave themselves that score and not less than that score.

3. Divide the group into three smaller groups.

▶ One group is to come up with ideas for supporting confidence; one group is to come up with ideas for supporting competence. Assure the groups that some ideas will come up in both groups and this is fine.

▶ The third group are to come up with practices to avoid and ways of destroying or undermining team members' confidence and competence.

▶ Give each group a sheet of A1 paper and some marker pens.

4. Show **Slide 4.11: Supporting confidence and competence** and, if necessary, prompt them with questions about their own personal experiences:

▶ What have people said to you that boosted your confidence?

▶ Past or present, how have other leaders or managers helped you grow your confidence and competence?

▶ What are you already doing to grow you team's competence?

▶ In an ideal situation, what would you like to do to support your team's confidence and competence?

For the third group these questions would be turned around and put in a negative manner eg "What can you do to crush your team's confidence?" or "What can you do to make people feel incompetent?"

Allow the small groups 15 minutes to complete this task.

5. When they begin their tasks, speak to each group in turn to make sure they understand the instructions and are on track.

After 15 minutes, call the groups back together.

6. Distribute **Handout 4.1: Supporting confidence and competence** and ask all participants to complete it during the feedback. They will do this by writing down:

   a. the ways that they already support their team's confidence and competence on the first page of the handout

   b. some ways to support their team's confidence and competence that they are willing to practise in the future on the second page

   c. ways of crushing confidence and competence that they will try to avoid on the third page.

This is a record of the ideas generated in this exercise for them to keep.

In turn, ask each group to speak about the ways they have discussed for supporting confidence, supporting competence and, as a lesson for what to avoid, for crushing confidence and competence. Ask each group to nominate a speaker who will describe what they have discussed. When this speaker has finished, ask if any other members of that group have any further ideas or contributions they wish to offer.

7. Finally, ask the remainder of the participants if they have any contributions to make.

Repeat this process for each group.

Allow 20 minutes for this feedback part of the exercise.

Points for the trainer

Although treating others as you would wish to be treated is a good rule of thumb it is still necessary to treat individuals as unique.

Exercise 4.2: Supporting values and meaning

Timing: 40 mins

Aims

▶ To remind participants of the Session 1 on values

▶ To brainstorm other ways that values and meaningfulness can be encouraged in others in their everyday work

Materials

▶ Slide 4.12: Three components of wholesome motivation (2)

▶ Slide 4.13: Values

▶ Slide 4.14: Supporting values and meaningfulness

▶ Handout 4.2: Supporting values and meaningfulness

▶ 3 X A1 sheets of flipchart paper

▶ marker pens

Notes for the trainer

1. Show *Slide 4.12: Three components of wholesome motivation (2)*.

▶ Explain that **Session 2: Personal Values** allowed participants to explore their values and, through this, how their work in health and care gains personal meaning. All team members will share the same human need for meaning in their work. Part of nurturing motivation among your team means supporting them in being clear about their values and finding ways of realising them in their work.

▶ The exercises done in Session 2 might be helpful for leaders to put into practice at work. However, they were classroom exercises and do require time and preparation. There are many other ways of helping to support values and meaning in your team. Many of you will be practising some of these already.

2. Show *Slide 4.13: Values* as a reminder of these exercises and, as appropriate, remind the group that they looked at:

    1. Writing about what you would like to hear said in your retirement speech

    2. Choosing values from a list

    3. How values are realised already in your day to day work

This is a brainstorming exercise using all your experience and all that you have learned from the past sessions, especially but not only, Session 2 (Values). The task is for you to come up with some practical ways of supporting values and meaningfulness for your frontline team.

3. Divide the group into three smaller groups:

▶ The first two groups are to come up with ideas for supporting values and meaningfulness for their teams

▶ The third group is to come up with practices to avoid and ways of destroying or undermining team members' values and meaningfulness at work

▶ Give each group a sheet of A1 paper and some marker pens.

Allow these small groups 15 minutes to complete this task. When they begin their tasks, speak to each group in turn to make sure they understand the instructions and are on track.

4. Show **Slide 4.14: Supporting values and meaningfulness** and, if necessary, prompt them with questions about their own personal experiences:

▶ What have people said that demonstrated the value of your work?

▶ Past or present, how have other leaders or managers helped understand how your work fits in with the broader values of the NHS or your work organisation or even of society at large?

▶ What are you already doing to make it clear to your team that their work makes a contribution?

▶ What can you do or say to help people persist with the boring, mundane or unpleasant aspects of their job?

Note: For the third group, these questions should be turned around and put in a negative manner eg "What could you do to diminish any sense of meaning for your team's work?"

Allow 15 minutes for this part of the exercise and then call the groups back together.

5. Give out **Handout 4.2: Supporting values and meaningfulness** and ask all participants to complete it during the feedback by writing down:

   a. the ways that they already support their team's values and sense of meaningfulness

   b. some ways to support their team's values and sense of meaningfulness that they are willing to practise in the future

   c. ways of crushing values and the sense of meaningfulness, which they will try to avoid.

This is a record of the ideas generated in this exercise for them to keep.

6. In turn ask each group to speak about the ways they have discussed for supporting values and a sense of meaningfulness, and, as a lesson for what to avoid, for crushing values and sense of meaningfulness.

▶ Ask each group to nominate a speaker who will describe what they have discussed. When this speaker has finished, ask if any other members of that group have any further ideas or contributions they wish to offer.

▶ Finally, ask the remainder of the participants if they have any contributions to make.

Points for the trainer

▶ Professional values are obligatory

▶ We can expect personal values to differ from person to person

▶ Showing people the value or the meaning of their work in the larger picture will help them get through mundane or difficult tasks

Exercise 4.3: Supporting a sense of belonging

Timing: 40 mins

Aims

▶ To explain how the concept of belonging is related to some of the more effective ways of using authority as discussed in Session 3, especially the use of referent power

▶ To expand on the idea of belongingness as being an important part of wholesome motivation

▶ To brainstorm ideas for ways to enhance a sense of belongingness in others in the participants' teams

Materials

▶ Slide 4.15: Three components of wholesome motivation (3)

▶ Slide 4.16: Belongingness

▶ Handout 4.3: Supporting a feeling of belongingness

▶ Handout 4.4: Supporting a feeling of belongingness – five top tips

▶ flipchart paper

▶ marker pens

Notes for the trainer

1. Show **Slide 4.15: Three components of wholesome motivation (3)**. The topic in Session 3 was the use of authority and this is relevant to supporting other's motivation, in the sense that all effective ways of using power will enhance a person's sense of belonging and being part of a team.

2. Show **Slide 4.16: Belongingness**.

▶ We will discuss the important idea of Belongingness, a fundamental human need. It is clear that feeling a valued member of the team or the work group is vital to sustained motivation. It is therefore an important part of the leader's role to ensure that all members of the team feel appreciated and that they belong.

▶ This, again, is a brainstorming exercise. Everybody present will have an idea of what it is like to feel a sense of belonging to a group. Also, most people will have an idea of what it is like not fitting in and to lack that sense of belonging.

▶ With particular, but not exclusive, reference to Session 3 that the use of some types of power is particularly effective at promoting a sense of belongingness, the task for the group is to come up with 'Five practical tips' for frontline leaders to support a sense of belonging in all their team members.

3. Give out **Handout 4.3: Supporting a feeling of belongingness**.

▶ Ask all participants to consider for a few minutes their own experiences of belongingness. Firstly, to think about a time and place when they felt a sense of belonging; secondly, to think about a time and place when they felt as if they did not fit in. In both cases they should write some notes on the handout about what others in those groups said and did that was relevant to that feeling.

▶ Ask participants to write these down in the first two boxes of Handout 4.3.

▶ If participants volunteer that there was a time when they did not feel as if they belonged to a group because they "did not live up to the team expectations" or something similar that reflects their own perceived personal failing, respond by asking again what was said or done by the other group members that resulted in that feeling.

Allow 5 minutes for this exercise.

4. Now ask the participants to get into pairs.

▶ The purpose of this part of the exercise is for the participants to talk over the notes they have made in the first part of the exercise and to compare them with the other person's. Ask them to discuss the similarities and differences.

Allow 10 minutes for this part of the exercise.

5. Ask each pair to split up depending upon whose surname comes first alphabetically and whose comes second. The 'first alphabetically' people will form one larger group and the 'second alphabetically' will form another.

▶ Give each of these groups a sheet of flipchart paper and some felt marker pens.

One group is tasked to produce a list of Five Top Tips of actions that leaders can take to ensure that a new member of staff will feel a sense of belonging to the team.

The other group is asked to produce a list of Five Top Tips of actions that leaders can take to ensure that current, maybe long-serving, members of the work team feel a sense of belonging.

▶ Ask the groups to decide on their top five tips and to write them down on the flipchart paper.

Allow 15 minutes for this part of the exercise.

6. Bring the two groups back in to the larger group and distribute **Handout 4.4: Supporting a feeling of belongingness – five top tips**.

▶ Ask for feedback from the two groups in turn. When each group has reported their Five Top Tips ask the other group if they have any comments or anything to add.

▶ Ask all participants to note down the Five Top Tips from each group on their copy of Handout 4.4 for their future use.

Points for the trainer

▶ By belonging, we feel as if we are part of something bigger and more important than ourselves.

▶ When people feel they belong to a group they will adopt the standards of behaviour of that group. This is a great way of attaining the observance of high standards.

Session summary

▶ Slide 4.17: Four components of good care leadership

▶ Slide 4.18: Three aspects of motivation

▶ Slide 4.19: Three components of wholesome motivation (4)

This is a quick reminder of the contents of the session, how they relate to each other and to the course as a whole.

Notes for the trainer

1. Show *Slide 4.17: Four components of good care leadership*.

Remind participants that this session on motivating others is one part of learning how to be an effective frontline leader and builds on the previous three sessions. The earlier sessions were largely about their self-development as a leader. This session has been how to develop their teams. All they have learned from Sessions 1 and 2 are directly applicable to motivating others. The learning from Session 3 was that the use of some types of power are particularly effective at promoting a sense of belongingness. We have expanded on this during this session.

2. Show *Slide 4.18: Three aspects of motivation*.

Remind participants that some staff may show a lack of motivation, and this may be their response to their work environment, or it may be a personal matter for them, or it may be a bit of both. It certainly is a problem and needs attention. There is also 'junk food' motivation, either to do with external rewards and punishments (carrots and sticks) or driven by the inner critic. Both are forms of motivation. Better still is 'wholesome' motivation which springs from within, is strong, resilient and persistent.

3. Show *Slide 4.19: Three components of wholesome motivation (4)*.

▶ Remind participants of the distinction made between 'junk food motivation' and 'wholesome motivation'; also, of the three components of wholesome motivation. These are three basic human needs that are always present for all of us and their satisfaction results in a powerful motivation that springs from within. We reflected that you cannot make somebody be motivated from within, you can only support their potential for inner motivation.

▶ Remind the group that they brainstormed these three components and they have written notes on what they can do in their workplace to support wholesome motivation.

4. Finally, thank the group for their participation and their contributions. Ask if they have any further questions.

Session 5: Project – Putting It Into Practice

Before the session

Arrangements should be made for some form of feedback from the project work that the group is planning to undertake.

The preferred way of doing this is to call another meeting of this group after 8–12 weeks. This would allow time for the projects to be undertaken. At this next meeting, each workgroup would be able to present their project, explain what they achieved and what they learned with a special focus on Confidence, Competence, Values, Use of Authority and Motivating Others.

The date and time for this reporting back meeting should be arranged with full management support before Session 5 is delivered.

Timing: 2hrs 30 mins

Overview

Small work groups will plan and commit to a project over the next few weeks. The project will take what they have learned in the previous four sessions and link it with the particular needs of their workplace. The project will be a practice in good care, one that is a small challenge but definitely manageable.

Activity	Time required
Introduction to the session	10 mins
Introduction to the project	20 mins
Writing project plans	1 hour 20 mins
Presenting project plans	40 mins

Materials

▶ Slides 5.1 to 5.7.

▶ Handouts 5.1 and 5.2

▶ A1 flipchart

▶ pens

Introduction to the session

Timing: 10 mins

Aims

▶ To welcome participants to the training day

▶ To inform them of the programme for the day

Materials

▶ Slide 5.1: Welcome

▶ Slide 5.2: Programme

Notes for the trainer

1. Show *Slide 5.1: Welcome*

▶ Welcome learners to the training day, introducing yourself and giving participants some background information about yourself as appropriate.

▶ Outline housekeeping arrangements, such as the procedure in the event of a fire, the mobile phone policy and the location of toilets etc.

2. Show *Slide 5.2: Programme*. Inform participants that the majority of the time today will be devoted to them writing their project plans in small work groups. Before that there will be a brief introduction to plan writing and at the end of the session they will be expected to present their plan to the larger group.

Tell the group that there is a reporting back meeting scheduled (give date, time and location) at which they will have the opportunity to feedback on their project. Stress that attendance at this meeting is an important part of the course. It will not be simply an occasion for celebration, although hopefully it will be that too. Feedback, lessons learned, obstacles overcome and so on are all highly relevant in the process of learning. Learning not only from our own experience but also from the experience of others.

Introduction to the project

Timing: 20 mins

Aims

▶ To explain clearly to the participants the nature of the task they are being set

▶ To explain how this project is designed to take the classroom learning from the 'Good Care Leadership' course into their day to day work

Materials

▶ Slide 5.3: Your project will…

▶ Slide 5.4: Your project may…

▶ Slide 5.5: When thinking about a project (1)

▶ Slide 5.6: When thinking about a project (2)

▶ Slide 5.7: When thinking about a project (3)

▶ Handout 5.1: Our project

▶ Handout 5.2: A worked example project

Everything that has been learned so far is of little use unless it is acted upon.

Notes for the trainer

1. Show **Slide 5.3 Your project will…**

Explain that good care leadership is demonstrated both in what you do, and also in the way you do it. So, when you are choosing a project bear this in mind. Your project is not expected to be world-changing. It is simply an exercise in good care (essential) and carried out in a way that will do at least two of the following:

▶ Help grow your confidence

▶ Help grow your competence

▶ Express or realise your values

▶ Involve the use of a type of authority

▶ Help to motivate others in your team

2. Show **Slide 5.4 Your project may…**

▶ Explain that projects should aim to be quite modest. Advise people not to over-reach by taking on a project that is possibly going to fail. The level to aim for is a small challenge, a challenge that will stretch the group members but is highly likely to succeed.

▶ Say this could be through a project related to the general 'culture' of the workplace, an educational innovation or it could be a direct patient-centred project.

▶ Within those limits the participants are free to choose their own projects to work on.

▶ Explain that the project may be quite small. If a group proposes a huge project suggest that they break it down into smaller units and only attempt the first stage for the present. They may move on to the larger project later.

3. Ask the group to form into work teams. Each team should be between two and six members. It is important to get people together who work in the same unit (ward, care home, clinic etc). It may be helpful to have a mix of disciplines but this is not essential. If, for example, a group of nurses wish to work together on a nursing related project and can justify it, that is fine. Sometimes the workgroups will emerge naturally but sometimes there will be a need for some direction from the trainer.

▶ Encourage people to be open minded about who they work with. Try to encourage people to work alongside people other than their best friends. Encourage diversity.

▶ Allow for some flexibility here as it is possible that people may wish to change work groups when the topics for projects are decided upon.

4. Give each participant a copy of **Handout 5.1: Our project**.

5. Show **Slide 5.5: When thinking about a project (1)**

Say that when thinking about their project, participants should consider both:

▶ their strengths (confidence, competence, values and authority)

▶ what their ward, care home, clinic or work unit needs.

6. Explain that both of these need to be kept in balance. It would be little use doing a project that had no relevance to the ward's or care home's needs. At the same time, it is important that the skills and knowledge learned in this course are used and practised. Whilst it is important to keep in mind the strengths of the team as a whole it is equally important not to pick a project that is simply a reflection of the team's special interests. There must be some clear benefit to the ward, care home or clinic.

7. Show **Slide 5.6 When thinking about a project (2)**

▶ Suggest that, to come up with ideas, you could ask yourself what is it about your current workplace that frustrates or annoys you or others? What do you see that is outdated or even poor practice? What do you hear patients and their relatives complain about? What do other staff complain about?

▶ Another way of stimulating ideas for a project would be for you to ask yourself the question, "If a real hotshot was employed in your place of work, took a look around and saw what was going on, what would she do?"

8. Remind participants that in **Exercise 2.3: Realising my values in my current work** they wrote notes about two of their chosen values and how they could improve the way that they live that value by making tiny steps in the right direction.

9. Show **Slide 5.7: When thinking about a project (3)**

▶ Ask participants if they recognise this scale. It is the scale that was used in the Session 1 exercise "How am I so wonderful?" This scale can be used for rating workplaces as well as people.

▶ Repeat the instructions for its use. Ask participants to allot a rating for their workplace between 0 and 10, between Completely Useless and Practically Perfect. Ask them not to spend too much time allotting a score; if there is disagreement they could go for a mid-point. The important points are:

▶ What happens on the ward/care home that makes the score, for example, 5 and not 4 or even 3? What is being *done well*, what is *going right*? Ask participants to generate a list of at least 10 instances or examples to illustrate this.

▶ Now, ask themselves, what could be done that would make the score a 6? (Insist that you do not want any ideas for making the score a 7 or higher. Small steps are all that is needed).

Writing project plans

Timing: 1 hr 20 mins

Aims

▶ For all participants to become part of a smaller group of colleagues from their own ward, care home or clinic. These workgroups will write a project plan to address a need in their workplace

▶ At the same time they will reflect upon how they are putting the skills and knowledge from the earlier four sessions of 'Good Care Leadership' into practice.

Materials

▶ Handout 5.1: Our project

▶ Handout 5.2: A worked example project

Notes for the trainer

1. At this point ask the small work groups to begin deciding on a subject for their project and then planning how to put it in to action.

2. Give out **Handout 5.1: Our project**

▶ Suggest that they have a good discussion about what they wish to work on for their project. Every person in the group should have a chance to have their say. Suggest that the quieter people use this as an opportunity to grow their confidence. Those who find it easy to take a lead should use the opportunity to pull back a little and practise a different style of using their influence.

▶ Go around all of the work groups to check that they fully understand the task. Answer any questions. If necessary, encourage ideas for project topics using open questions, elaborating on the questions in **Slide 5.6: When thinking about a project (2)** and **Slide 5.7: When thinking about a project (3)**. Do not suggest project topics for the workgroup, this is their responsibility.

3. When a work group has agreed on a topic, ask them to fill in the blank form describing their project using the following headings.

Title

Rationale

A few sentences on why this particular topic has been chosen. Indicate the need and the values that will be expressed in this project

Background

Here you can write a little more about the need, including any relevant statistics. You can describe any related previous interventions or projects.

Goal

A brief statement of the ultimate goal of your project.

All goals should be SMART.

- ▶ Specific – state clearly what you will do
- ▶ Measurable – how will you know when it is accomplished?
- ▶ Achievable – realistic within the constraints of your workplace
- ▶ Relevant – worthwhile and applicable
- ▶ Timed – can be achieved in time before the feedback meeting

Steps

Explicit descriptions of the actions that need to be taken to arrive at the goal. Best done in time order if applicable.

Timeline

A proposal for dates by which each step will be completed.

Resources

This might include material objects, time, management support, budget.

Constraints

Anything that might be or become an obstacle to completing the project. This can vary from going over budget to bad weather for an outdoor event.

Responsibilities

Allocate each step to an individual or individuals to ensure accountability.

Link to the Good Care Leadership components

Ask each group to write an explanation of how their project will impact on the four components of this course. This is important and will be a strong stimulus to reflection. It is also something that can be revisited as the project progresses, especially when obstacles or difficulties are encountered.

4. Give out *Handout 5.2: A worked example project* and explain this is only an example that they may use as an illustration but need not be bound by.

Allow 1 hour 20 minutes for this exercise.

Presenting project plans

Timing: 40 mins

Aim

▶ For all workgroups to have the opportunity to present their project to the wider group, to explain what workplace needs will be met and what it is from the 'Good Care Leadership' course that they will be practising

Notes for the trainer

1. Call all participants back together into the larger group. Ask each workgroup in turn to give a brief presentation of their project plan. Encourage questions and suggestions as appropriate. It is important to keep an eye on timing here to ensure that all groups have sufficient time to speak about their plans.

Ending

When all presentations have been made thank the group for their participation and for their work in writing project plans.

Remind them of the arrangements for reporting back and wish them luck with their projects.

PowerPoint slides

Session 1: Confidence and Competence

Slide 1.1: Welcome

Slide 1.2: Programme

Slide 1.3: Four components of good care leadership

Slide 1.4: Ways of viewing confidence 1

Slide 1.5: Ways of viewing confidence 2

Slide 1.6: False confidence and true confidence

Slide 1.7: Discuss a time I was…

Slide 1.8: What have I achieved?

Slide 1.9: Three challenges

Slide 1.10: Perfect v Useless 1

Slide 1.11: Perfect v Useless 2

Slide 1.12: Parts of leadership

Slide 1.13: A continuum

Slide 1.14: False confidence

Slide 1.15: Confidence varies

Slide 1.16: What have I achieved?

Slide 1.17: What have I achieved?

Slide 1.18: A good leader

Slide 1.19: How am I so wonderful?

Session 2: Personal values

Slide 2.1: Welcome

Slide 2.2: Programme

Slide 2.3: Four components of good care leadership

Slide 2.4: Personal values (1)

Slide 2.5: Personal values (1)

Slide 2.6: Personal values (1)

Slide 2.7: Personal values (1)

Slide 2.8: Personal values (1)

Slide 2.9: Personal values (1)

Slide 2.10: Personal values (1)

Slide 2.11: Personal values (1)

Slide 2.12: Personal values (2)

Slide 2.13: My retirement speech

Slide 2.14: Examples

Slide 2.15: Examples

Slide 2.16: Parts of leadership

Slide 2.17: The nature of values

Slide 2.18: Retirement speech

Slide 2.19: List of values

Slide 2.20: Values in action

Slide 2.21: Personal values (3)

Session 3: Use of Authority

Slide 3.1: Welcome

Slide 3.2 Programme

Slide 3.3: Four components of good care leadership

Slide 3.4: Ward culture

Slide 3.5: Culture change

Slide 3.6: The power of the individual

Slide 3.7: Legitimate/positional power

Slide 3.8: Using legitimate/positional power

Slide 3.9: Reward power

Slide 3.10: Using reward power

Slide 3.11: Coercive power

Slide 3.12: Using coercive power

Slide 3.13: Expert power

Slide 3.14: Using expert power

Slide 3.15: Referent power

Slide 3.16: Using referent power

Slide 3.17: Moral challenges

Slide 3.18: Using your authority

Slide 3.19: Using your authority

Slide 3.20: Using your authority

Slide 3.21: Using your authority

Slide 3.22: Using your authority

Slide 3.23: Using your authority

Slide 3.24: Using your authority

Slide 3.25: Using your authority

Session 4: Motivating others

Slide 4.1: Welcome

Slide 4.2: Programme

Slide 4.3: Four components of good care leadership

Slide 4.4: Complete lack of motivation

Slide 4.5: Junk food motivation (1)

Slide 4.6: Junk food motivation (2)

Slide 4.7: Wholesome motivation (1)

Slide 4.8: Wholesome motivation (2)

Slide 4.9: Three components of wholesome motivation (1)

Slide 4.10: Confidence and competence

Slide 4.11: Supporting confidence and competence

Slide 4.12: Three components of wholesome motivation (2)

Slide 4.13: Values

Slide 4.14: Supporting values and meaningfulness

Session 5: Project – Putting It Into Practice

Handouts

Handout 1.1: Discuss a time I was…

Handout 1.2: What have I achieved, so far?

Handout 1.3: Three challenges

Handout 1.4: A good leader I have known

Handout 1.5: How am I so wonderful?

Handout 2.1: Your own retirement speech

Handout 2.2: Choosing your own values

Handout 2.3a: Values in your daily work

Handout 2.3b: Values in your daily work

Handout 3.1: A clinical case study

Handout 3.2: Legitimate or positional power

Handout 3.3: Reward power

Handout 3.4: Coercive power

Handout 3.5: Expert power

Handout 3.6: Referent power

Handout 3.7: Using legitimate/positional power

Handout 3.8: Using reward power

Handout 3.9: Using coercive power

Handout 3.10: Using expert power

Handout 3.11: Using referent power

Handout 4.1: Supporting confidence and competence

Handout 4.2: Supporting values and meaningfulness

Handout 4.3: Supporting a feeling of belongingness

Handout 4.4: Supporting a feeling of belongingness – five top tips

Handout 5.1: Our project

Handout 5.2: A worked example project

Theory and Evidence

Introduction

The exercises presented here are intended to be straightforward and accessible to all. Yet they have been carefully designed and are intended to build on a lot of background work from scholars in several branches of psychology, nursing and management studies. There is a lot of thinking going on 'under the bonnet'. Anybody who is interested may follow up the theory and the evidence behind Good Care Leadership through the selected readings given below. Readings are suggested for each of the first four sessions but first of all there are some readings that have helped me understand why the practice of good care is so very difficult.

The problem of poor care

Although the Good Care Leadership course does not teach about the causes of poor care, it is based on an analysis that attributes much to difficult working conditions. Three major aspects are:

▶ The high levels of stress, both physical and emotional, that are common in care work

▶ Being pulled in two directions when governance demands are prioritised over care tasks

▶ The social psychology of the workgroup that can, under certain circumstances, lead good people to behave in bad ways

1. Stress

Everybody knows that work overload is exhausting. The sheer amount of physical labour and the number of tasks required to be performed each working day can be overwhelming. Moreover, in care work this physical stress is compounded by psychological challenges. The particular demands of working with sick people are discussed in Pam Smith's work on Emotional Labour. Illness, dying and distress are everyday occurrences in this work. Furthermore, we know that not all patients are polite and cooperative and can sometimes be extremely challenging. Working in these conditions is wholly unlike working in an office and is very highly emotionally demanding.

Smith P (1992) *The Emotional Labour of Nursing*. London: Macmillan.

Persaud R (2004) Faking it: The emotional labour of medicine. *British Medical Journal* **329** (6) 87.

Gray B and Smith P (2009) Emotional labour and the clinical settings of nursing care. *Nurse Education in Practice* **9** (4) 253–61.

One example of how stress affects professionals' behaviour comes from a mixed method study of hospital ward nurses. This revealed that, when they are prevented by overwork from giving good quality care, they sometimes develop an unusual way of coping with their frustration. Instead of giving all patients equal but unsatisfactory care, some nurses lavish time and attention on their 'favourite' patients. Naturally, this is to the detriment of the care given to other patients. One may see that this is inequitable, but it does allow those nurses the satisfaction of knowing that in this difficult environment they have managed to give decent care to at least one person.

Maben J, Adams M, Peccei R et al (2012) "Poppets and parcels". *International Journal of Older People Nursing* **7** (2) 83–94.

2. Being pulled in two directions

Care staff are supposed to care, health and care organisations claim that providing top quality care is their mission. Yet too often care staff are required to prioritise non-care duties. These could be attending meetings, completing returns, ordering supplies, tidying the laundry cupboard, teaching and so on. None of these are bad in themselves, it is just a matter of priorities. When non-care duties are routinely prioritised over care tasks there is the risk of demoralising frontline staff. A classic description of what happens when organisations claim to be promoting one thing but are effectively rewarding another is provided in:

Kerr S (1975) On the folly of rewarding A while hoping for B. *Academy of Management Journal* **18** (4) 769–783.

This paper is relevant to Session 3: Use of Authority in which we discuss the role of reward power and its limitations. It is also relevant to Session 4 where external rewards are considered part of 'junk food motivation'.

3. The social psychology of groups

Overwork and inappropriate demands may seriously affect morale or even lead to burnout. But to explain some of the excesses of neglect and even cruelty that have hit the headlines in recent years we need to dig deeper into human psychology. Two landmark studies stand out.

Stanley Milgram's work on obedience to authority experiments shocked the world by showing just how easy it is to persuade ordinary people to act in a way that is harmful to others. In his experiments, this meant asking ordinary people to administer increasingly severe electric shocks (the shocks were faked, nobody was harmed). This was surprisingly easy, with 65% of participants administering shocks they believed to be severe and dangerous. Modern interpretations suggest that people may allow their usual ethical standards to be overridden if they can be persuaded to accept an alternative justification, something that appeals to a 'greater good'.

The original report can be found in:

Milgram S (1963) Behavioral study of obedience. *Journal of Abnormal and Social Psychology* **67** (4) 371–378.

There is also plenty of material including videos available online, for example

www.simplypsychology.org/milgram.html (accessed November 2020)

Philip Zimbardo set up a fake prison and randomly allocated student volunteers to be either 'guards' or 'prisoners'. The experiment was set to last a fortnight but had to be stopped after 6 days due to the abuse being practised by the 'guards'. This is a particularly strong example of the effect of intergroup hostility. The lesson from this, and also from decades of social psychological research, is that if you divide people into Them and Us with a difference in power between the two groups, there is a very real risk of hostility and harm towards the weaker group. Intergroup hostility is considered to be the psychological basis for bias, discrimination, stereotyping and genocide. Hospital wards and care homes are places where two groups, staff and patients/residents, exist with a great power imbalance.

The original report of the Stanford Prison Experiment can be found in:

Haney S, Banks C and Zimbardo P (1973) A study of prisoners and guards in a simulated prison. *Naval Research Reviews* **9**, 1–17.

Zimbardo also provides extra information at the www.prisonexp.org/the-story/ accessed November 2020

After a career of studying wicked behaviour, Zimbardo is now involved with the more positive side of human nature: www.heroicimagination.org

A more recent take on interpreting the factors at work in the Milgram and Zimbardo experiments is found in:

Haslam SA and Reicher SD (2012) Contesting the "Nature" Of Conformity: *PLoS Biology* **10**(11).

An examination of the relevance of this research to real life problems is given in:

Fiske ST, Harris LT, Cuddy AJC (2004) Why ordinary people torture enemy prisoners. *Science* (306), 1482–1483.

The puzzle of why more staff do not object to poor practice may be at least partially answered by consideration of the 'Bystander Effect', a remarkably resilient phenomena in which the likelihood of an individual stepping in to halt harm to a vulnerable person decreases the more people present:

Darley JM and Latane B (1968) Bystander intervention in emergencies: Diffusion of responsibility. *Journal of Personality and Social Psychology* **8** (4p1) 377.

The papers above highlight the strength of the situation in determining human behaviour, primarily in eliciting evil behaviour. The other side of the coin is the relative weakness of individual characteristics (like honesty and courage) in determining behaviour:

Doris JD (2002) *Lack of Character: Personality and moral behaviour.* Cambridge University Press.

4. The hope for good care

The Milgram and Zimbardo studies may result in us feel pessimistic about human nature and the way people are so strongly affected by the situations. Yet there is also good evidence that individuals and minority groups are not always crushed by the majority. Conformity and inter group hostility are not inevitable. There is a school of study of Small Group Influence that demonstrates how like-minded people can act together to bring about change.

Moscovici SE, Mucchi-Faina AE and Maass AE (1994) *Minority Influence*. Nelson-Hall Publishers.

There is also evidence of nurses in leadership positions providing excellent care in situations where others all around them are failing.

For example, the case of "An impoverished Trust, an enriched ward" is described in some detail in Section 7 of:

Patterson M, Nolan M, Rik J et al (2011) *From Metrics to Meaning: Culture Change and Quality of Acute Hospital Care for Older People*. Report for the National Institute for Health Research Service. NIHR SDO programme project, 3(1501), 93. Retrieved on 10 August 2020 from: http://www.netscc.ac.uk/hsdr/files/project/SDO_FR_08-1501-93_V01.pdf

Patterson *et al* describe an NHS Trust that is performing poorly in many ways. Yet one ward stands out as being excellent and renowned for its high quality of patient care.

In this paper credit for the excellent care delivered on the ward is entirely given to the ward manager. The paper considers her leadership style which some people may find helpful.

In summary, both the character of the individual and the situation they find themselves in play important roles in determining moral and caring behaviour. Furthermore, both interact with each other in dynamic ways. One possible result is a vicious circle of poor 'culture', poor care, leading to staff demoralisation and hopelessness with further destructive effects on the quality of care offered and the resulting culture. Good staff leave and those who are prepared to tolerate lower standards stay. Poor care does not appear out of nowhere but takes time to develop.

The other possibility is a virtuous circle in which a high-quality culture assures good quality care. The staff are empowered and motivated which leads to further improvements in care quality. Good staff queue up to work here. This seems obvious, but we need to bear in mind two considerations. The first is the unexpected power of situations to crush good intentions. Anybody seeking to change a poor culture has a very difficult job on their hands and would be well advised to seek as many allies as they can. The second is that the desire to provide compassionate care is a delicate plant and itself needs care and a nurturing environment.

Session 1: Confidence and Competence

People make judgements of how well they will be able to do certain tasks or deal with certain situations and these judgements may be only loosely connected to their actual abilities. People who have a high (but not unrealistic) view of their own capabilities and competences are more likely to take on difficult tasks and challenges, are motivated to persist longer in difficult tasks and generally turn in a higher performance at work. People who judge themselves as less capable tend to avoid difficult tasks, are more easily discouraged and generally perform less well at work.

The rationale for encouraging people to call to mind their achievements in the exercises is that these are all factors that positively affect confidence in their competence. The key reference is:

Bandura A (1982) Self efficacy mechanism in human agency. *American Psychologist* **37** (2) 122–147.

The graph on Slide 1.6 is a representation of the "Dunning-Kruger effect". There is a rather dry and theoretical description of it on Wikipedia and this is mostly concerned with the early peak of unwarranted over-confidence at the beginning of a job or project. Many readers will have been there and fallen into the 'trough of despair'. It is used in this course to illustrate that even after falling into a 'trough of despair' self-confidence can be regained over time. This is done through a proper assessment of their real capabilities.

Session 2: Personal Values

Leaders are in a position of power over others. It is essential that they use this power in a way that is ethically appropriate. Power should be exercised for the benefit of their patients, their staff, the organisation they work for and for society at large. It should not be exercised solely for personal benefit.

There are two main sources of support for the clear articulation of personal values to increase motivation and effort at work. The first comes from social psychological studies of underperformance by certain minority groups who are stereotyped as being 'naturally' less capable at learning certain subjects. A 15-minute exercise of writing down one's most deeply held values was trialled with a group of women studying a physics course. This intervention was sufficient to significantly reduce the achievement gap with their male colleagues. This study can be found in:

Miyake A, Kost-Smith LE, Finkelstein, ND et al (2010) Reducing the gender achievement gap in college science: a classroom study of values affirmation. *Science* **330** (6008) 1234–1237.

A summary of wider applications is available in:

Cohen GL and Sherman DK (2014) The psychology of change: self-affirmation and social psychological intervention. *Annual Review of Psychology* **65**(1) 333–371.

The second source comes from Acceptance and Commitment Therapy (ACT). The emphasis that ACT places on Values puts the patients' problems in the context of what sort of person they want to be and the life they wish to lead. This way the solution to a problem can be approached through the way that it interferes with a person's values. So, agoraphobia might be approached in the way that it interferes with the wish to be a good parent. By bringing the value of wishing to be a good parent to the fore, ACT therapists find that they can harness the patients' own motivation, in this case taking their child out to the park, to school and to other outdoor activities. The force of motivation linked to realising values can be very strong and sufficient to help people overcome serious problems. There are many ACT resources online. There are two particularly good introductory texts:

Hayes SC (2005) *Get Out of Your Mind and Into Your Life*. New Harbinger Publications.

Harris R (2007) *The Happiness Trap*. Constable Robinson Publications.

A real-life example from the nursing literature illustrates the importance of values and ideals in frontline clinical care. In this case, unfortunately, it shows the harm that is done when values are allowed to erode. The study describes the wearing down of values and idealism among newly qualified nurses. In particular, the authors draw our attention to the loss of ideals about compassionate care when the nurses are working on wards that are overstretched and poorly led. Under these conditions, the authors identified a set of 'covert rules' that replaced the new nurses' high ideals:

Maben J, Latter S and Macleod Clark J (2007) The sustainability of ideals, values and the nursing mandate: evidence from a longitudinal qualitative study. *Nursing Inquiry* **14** (2) 99–113.

Session 3: Power/Authority/Influence

The five sources of power are from:

French J, Raven B and Cartwright D (1959) The Bases of Social Power. *Classics of Organization Theory* **7**, 311–320.

A fuller discussion of these sources of power, along with a lengthy discussion of theories of power and influence methods can be found in:

Yukl G (2013) *Leadership in Organizations*. London: Pearson, Chapter 8.

The multiple ways of using power are discussed in a paper by the consulting firm the Hay Group. They found that among the senior ward nurses they studied, those who performed best were able to utilise a variety of what they referred to as different "Leadership Styles". These styles map loosely on to the sources of power identified by French & Raven but the point of the article is made in the title of the paper:

Hay Group (2007) Nurse Leadership: Being nice is not enough. https://www.networks. nhs.uk/nhs-networks/matrons-national-network/network-events/nurse_leadership.pdf/ view

One takes the point that it is necessary sometimes to coach, sometimes to be directive, sometimes to be firm as well as at times being 'nice'. Yet it is my feeling is that niceness, or, to use the psycho-jargon, empathy and interpersonal warmth, is a good starting point for any leader.

The Patterson *et al* paper mentioned above gives a pen portrait of the Ward Sister in charge of "An Enriched Ward" and clearly identifies many of the important aspects of her leadership style. She is capable of using a variety of sources of power, or leadership styles, according to what is necessary:

> 'It's very supportive but it's also, I guess it's a little bit authoritarian but that makes people work harder and try and meet standards that they need to be meeting."

Session 4: Motivating Others

Decades of research have shown very clearly that people perform best at work when they are motivated from within. That is, their drive to perform well comes from their strong personal identification with their role. They say things like, *"It is just the sort of person I am"*; or *"It's not special, it's just what you would expect a nurse to do"*. This contrasts with outcomes when managers attempt to motivate their workforce by using external rewards and punishments. Such efforts ensure that the worker's efforts are contractual and managers risk being seen as manipulative. Worse, rewarding acts that people are already doing due to their own inner motivation often leads to a diminution of that motivation and a worsening of performance when the rewards are removed. In general, external rewards lead to mere compliance and 'gaming'.

Intrinsic motivation leads to strong performance, greater effort, better problem solving, more persistence and higher levels of work satisfaction.

The science of motivation is complicated and I have collapsed the fourfold classification of types of motivation into two types, Junk Food and Wholesome motivation. Junk Food refers to external motivation through rewards and punishments and also to inner punitive motivation through a strict and anxious 'inner critic'. Wholesome motivation describes two sub-types. Intrinsic Motivation is when a task is simply inherently enjoyable or pleasing the way that play is to a child. Autonomous Internalised Motivation is when people are driven by the sense that their work has a certain value. This latter form of motivation is especially powerful. Seeing the meaning in one's work enables one to tolerate considerable boredom or difficulty in achieving it. As Neitzsche said, "He who has a why can bear any how".

There are two good papers explaining this field of research. The first is more theoretical and the second more practical.

Deci EL, Olafsen AH and Ryan RM (2017) Self-determination theory in work organizations: the state of a science. Annual Review of *Organizational Psychology and Organizational Behavior* **4** (1) 19–43.

Stone DN, Deci EL and Ryan RM (2008) Beyond talk: creating autonomous motivation through self-determination theory. *Journal of General Management* **34**(3) 75–91.

A similar concept of *meaningfulness* at work has been explored through interviews with people across a range of occupations (including nursing). The results show that the task of leaders is to create environments that nurture a sense of meaningfulness, and thus motivation, effort, commitment and satisfaction.

Bailey C and Madden A (2016) What makes work meaningful —or meaningless. *MIT Sloan Management Review*, 2016 (Summer) 53–61.

Links to other qualifications and standards

Skills for Care

The **Care Certificate** and Levels 3 & 4 Diplomas in Care contain units with the theme of Personal Development and Values.

The **Level 5 Diploma in Leadership and Management in Adult Care** units in the areas of DILMAC 1A & B, Leadership and Management, DILMAC 4A Relationships and partnership working, DILMAC 5C Continuous improvement, DILMAC 6A & B Professional development, supervision and performance management, DILMAC 9A Managing self.

The content of Good Care Leadership covers aspects of the following SfC modules:

▶ Leadership Qualities Framework: Demonstrating personal qualities; Working with others; Managing services (Managing people and managing performance); Improving services (Encouraging improvement, facilitating transformation)

▶ Managing People: Building resilience; Code of Conduct; Developing your staff; People performance; Supervision

▶ Transforming Care: Set the right culture and values; Workforce development

▶ Leadership Starts With Me – entire unit

The NHS Knowledge and Skills Framework dimensions

▶ Personal and people development

▶ Service Improvement

▶ Quality

The NHS Leadership Academy dimensions

▶ Inspiring shared purpose

▶ Leading with care

▶ Sharing the vision

▶ Engaging the team

▶ Holding to account

▶ Influencing for results

Registered Nurse revalidation

Good Care Leadership is particularly suited to the compulsory nursing revalidation process for all qualified nurses. As well as being a form of CPD, as a reflective development process it is an excellent basis for the requirements for written reflective accounts and the requirement to have had reflective discussions. The course is relevant to the NMC Code, Section 25 Leadership. The Values exercises directly relate to The NMC Code of ethical practice.

Handouts

All of the handouts in this section can be downloaded at
www.pavpub.com/good-care-leadership-resources

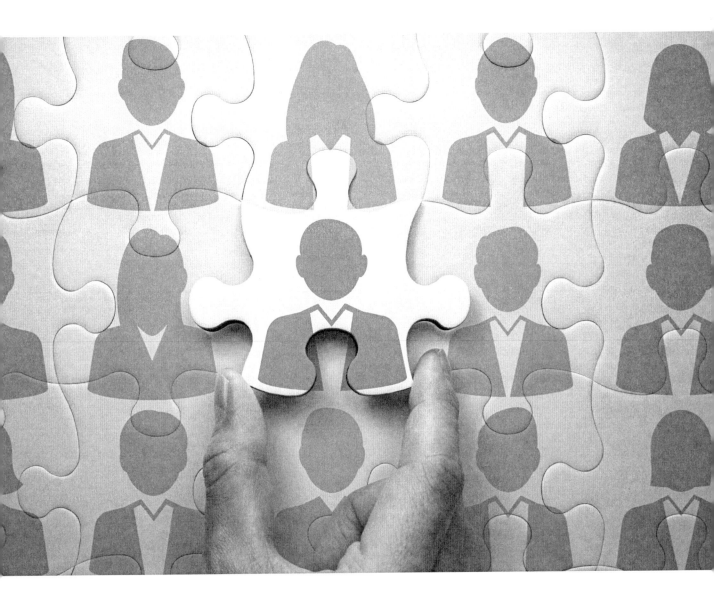

Handout 1.1: Discuss a time I was...

Feeling confident	Feeling unconfident
Briefly describe the situation or the event	Briefly describe the situation or the event
What factors influenced my feeling confident?	What factors influenced my feeling unconfident?

Handout 1.2: What have I achieved, so far?

Make a list of all your most important achievements.

This can include anything you consider an achievement – exams passed, qualifications gained, courses attended, skills mastered, knowledge gleaned. It might also include difficult tasks completed, people's needs attended to, problems or puzzles solved, challenges accepted.

Handout 1.3: Three challenges

Sometimes we can learn more about ourselves when we are under stress than we can when everything is running smoothly. Below you are asked to write some notes about times in your career when you had to face difficulties or challenges of some sort.

These do not have to be challenges that you have fully overcome. They may be things that continue to challenge you to this day.

Handout 1.4: A good leader I have known

This will be somebody you have known at work. An 'everyday' leader, not a 'great' man or woman.

Their initials   Their official position

What did this person do or say to make them a good leader?

What did you learn from this person?

How would you apply what you have learned in your practice?

Handout 1.5: How am I so wonderful?

1. Assign yourself a score as a professional on the scale below.

| 0 | | 2 | | 4 | | 6 | | 8 | | 10 |

COMPLETELY
USELESS

PRACTICALLY
PERFECT

2. Discuss with a colleague all the reasons why you are so good as the score that you
have given yourself. What is it about you that gives you this score? What talents,
knowledge and skills do you have, what do you do that makes you this score rather
than a score one or two points below it? List all these attributes below.

Handout 2.1: Your own retirement speech

In this exercise you are asked to imagine you are about to hear a speech given in celebration of you at your retirement.

Please note below the most important things about you and your work that you would really like to hear spoken about.

Handout 2.2: Choosing your own values

From the list below, choose the values that you think are important to you.

Mark them according to how important they are to you.

▶ This value is very important to me – put a circle around five values

▶ This value is moderately important to me – underline these

▶ This value is not important to me – leave these unmarked

Wisdom	Patience	Order	Mindfulness	Independence
Humility	Flexibility	Gratitude	Safety	Forgiveness
Spirituality	Responsibility	Power	Challenge	Encouragement
Adventure	Intimacy	Pleasure	Romance	Connection
Curiosity	Loyalty	Beauty	Skillfulness	Sexuality
Self-control	Self-development	Self-care	Self-awareness	Supportiveness
Respect	Reciprocity	Open mindedness	Fun	Contribution
Thoughtfulness	Tolerance	Assertiveness	Caring	Authenticity
Cooperation	Conformity	Compassion	Equality	Creativity
Excitement	Fairness	Fitness	Freedom	Friendliness
Generosity	Honesty	Justice	Courage	Humour
Sensuality	Love	Knowledge	Kindness	

Handout 2.3a: Values in your daily work

Write down your top five values in the first column below.

In the second column write down what you do in your daily work that show that you are living and working to this value.

NOTE: Please only write what you *do*. Not what you think or feel or wish. In this exercise we are looking for actions or words, things that would be seen or heard if somebody was recording you with a video camera.

Value	What you already do to realise this value?

Handout 2.3b: Values in your daily work

Write down your chosen two values in the first column below.

In the second column write down what you will do in your daily work that will make this value more evident.

NOTE: Please only write what you will do. Not what you will think or feel or wish. In this exercise we are looking for actions or words, things that would be seen or heard if somebody was recording you with a video camera.

Value	What small change can you make to realise this value even more?

Handout 3.1: A clinical case study

I am rostered for one shift per week only, but I am counted in the numbers for the shift so I'm not supernumerary. I, and the managers who work under me, all try to give positive verbal and written feedback to staff for good work done and to mention it in staff meetings and the monthly newsletter.

I have no doubt that some staff at some times will say horrible things about the way I work and what I do. That goes with the territory and doesn't bother me. I believe that giving praise to people for working hard and doing well ***is the right thing to do*** *(her emphasis)*. It's not a management ploy, or a 'tactic' to get people to work harder. Neither is it about trying to be popular. It's about human-being-to-human-being respect and valuing colleagues as whole people who bring their whole selves to their jobs and give of themselves every day.

My belief is, and I might be horribly deluded, that staff here appreciate being praised and thanked. They seem to, and say so, and more importantly, they praise and thank others (I hear it happening all the time, not directed by me). But they know I mean it. And maybe congruence is the core of this. I hope the staff I work with know that when they get a letter from me they can trust it, because they see me in action every day and, most of the time, I act in the same way. That is, positive about them, respectful towards them, never slagging anyone off to them and never slagging them off to anyone else. I protect their interests as best I can and those of our patients. I leap to every staff member's defence in public (even if I then tear them off a strip in private). I genuinely believe that all our staff do a fantastic job in so many ways. I don't have to put that on, it's true to me. I guess part of them trusting me is that I am out there with them. I do shifts, on calls, come in in the middle of the night, go to home visits. As someone said to me recently, 'We know you would never ask us to do anything that you would not do yourself.'

I take my responsibility for the service very seriously, but I do try to share decision-making. We have had quite a few ballots on issues, where all staff have got to 'vote' on a matter. Other decisions are thrashed out at meetings. Occasionally, I think there are decisions that just have to be made and I'm happy to do that. It's not a brilliant strategy though and can go horribly wrong. Because I do it so rarely people get very shocked and upset when I do it!

I think I did say that part of a manager's job is to protect staff from stress. For me this is about fighting battles with the next layer up.

Handout 3.2: Legitimate or positional power

This is the power that comes with the holding of a position of formal authority. It is usually explicitly stated in official documents and is also widely accepted as a norm within the organisation.

Legitimate power can be backed up with organisational sanctions up to disciplinary procedures and sacking. Usually, things do not go that far because of its widespread acceptance. The extent of a person's positional power is usually defined in organisational documents, such as job descriptions.

Using legitimate or positional power

▶ Be respectful

▶ Make polite requests

▶ Give reasons for your requests

▶ Ensure requests are clear, written if necessary

▶ Follow up and remind if necessary

▶ Follow proper channels

▶ Verify compliance

▶ Insist on compliance, as appropriate

Handout 3.3: Reward power

This is the power that comes with people knowing, or believing, that you control important rewards. It is unusual for frontline health and care leaders to have much discretion over monetary and other tangible rewards. Yet they may be able to give or withhold other rewards such as a good reference, better work schedules, opportunities for job development and training.

Above all, they have at their disposal attention, praise and recognition for a job well done. Not all rewards are tangible and many of the most effective are social in their nature.

Using reward power

▶ Be fair and ethical – do not have favourites

▶ Link rewards to specific actions

▶ Ensure rewards are valued

▶ Give praise that is appropriate to the individual

▶ Look out for good work, show that you notice it

▶ Praise much more than you criticise

▶ Be genuine, do not offer praise 'on a rota'

Handout 3.4: Coercive power

This is the power to inflict some sort of punishment or pressure on people. Mostly this will relate to your junior staff, but not always. This may be officially sanctioned, for example formal disciplinary procedures. No organisation would want to be without serious sanctions in extreme situations.

But coercive power is also used informally as reprimands that can vary from a frown to a full dressing down. A 'punishment' is *anything* the recipient finds unpleasant. Therefore, many ways of expressing disapproval can be used to steer behaviour when necessary.

"That's not the way we do it here" or

"You could have done better"

Be aware that the use of coercive power will generally result in compliance and only rarely in full commitment. It may also result in resentment and opposition.

Using coercive power

▶ Ensure that standards and requirements are clear and well known

▶ Respond swiftly to lapses

▶ Criticise the behaviour not the person eg "That was the wrong thing to do" rather than "You are a stupid/lazy/bad person"

▶ Reprimand in private if possible

▶ Best used sparingly

▶ Accompany with showing how to improve performance

▶ Follow up on warnings

Handout 3.5: Expert power

The possession of knowledge, skills or expertise, especially if these are rare and valued, can confer much power on the holder. People who know the best way to perform a procedure or deal with a particular issue and who are up to date with professional developments will have more power than those who do not.

This knowledge must be relevant to the work situation and the influence it confers will be limited to this area of expertise.

It may be necessary to demonstrate that this expertise is both important and not easily available from other sources.

Using expert power

▶ You may need to show that your expertise is relevant and that it is not easily available elsewhere

▶ You must know your stuff and stay up to date

▶ Speak confidently, but do not bluff

▶ Do not lecture other people

▶ Acknowledge others' knowledge and opinions, few people are totally ignorant even in your area of expertise

▶ Admit the limits of your expertise and do not overstep them

Handout 3.6: Referent power

Stems from people's desire to please or emulate a person who they admire, trust and respect and who they feel is 'on their side'. The reasons for this might be a recognition of their clinical excellence, their high standards or their concern for their patients and staff. All clinical leaders will possess some of these qualities to some degree. Not everybody can be Florence Nightingale but we can all aim to stimulate respect and loyalty from our teams. Naturally, referent power may be totally independent of formal position and reward or coercive power.

You may feel that this does not apply to you, that your team take no notice of you. In fact, they will be watching you all the time.

Using referent power

▶ Being a consistent role model

▶ Showing concern for your team

▶ Regarding them positively and showing it

▶ Behaving with integrity, acting your values

▶ Appreciating their values

▶ Persisting in all this over time

Handout 3.7: Using legitimate/positional power

This is the power that comes with the holding of a position of formal authority. It is usually explicitly stated in official documents and is also widely accepted as a norm within the organisation. Legitimate power can be backed up with organisational sanctions up to disciplinary procedures and sacking. Usually things do not go that far because of its widespread acceptance. The extent of a person's positional power is usually defined in organisational documents, such as job descriptions.

	Mostly	Sometimes	Rarely	Comfortable Y/N
I make polite requests rather than abrupt commands				
I explain the reasons for requests that I make				
I use language that is clear and comprehensible when making a request				
In emergency situations I am firm and assertive				
In non-emergency situations I am polite but firm and confident				
Complex requests are written down as necessary so they are fully understood and not forgotten				
I follow up and check on orders and requests to ensure compliance				
When necessary I insist on compliance				

Handout 3.8: Using reward power

The power that comes with people knowing, or believing, that you control important rewards. It is unusual for frontline healthcare leaders to have much discretion over monetary and other tangible rewards. Yet they may be able to give or withhold other rewards such as a good reference, better work schedules, opportunities for job development.

Above all, we have at our disposal praise and recognition for a job well done. Not all rewards are tangible and many of the most effective are social in their nature.

	Mostly	Sometimes	Rarely	Comfortable Y/N
I offer rewards (eg approval) in a manner that is appropriate to the person				
I do not show favouritism when offering rewards				
I do not promise more than I can give				
I explain the specific reason for giving rewards				
I notice and acknowledge people who are giving that bit extra				
I give praise far more often than I give criticism				
I find out (and reward) what people are doing right				

Handout 3.9: Using coercive power

This is the power to inflict some sort of punishment or pressure on people. Mostly this will relate to your junior staff, but not always. This may be officially sanctioned, for example formal disciplinary procedures. No organisation would want to be without serious sanctions in extreme situations.

But coercive power is also used informally as reprimands that can vary from a frown to a full dressing down. A 'punishment' is anything the recipient finds unpleasant. Therefore, many ways of expressing disapproval can be used to steer behaviour when necessary.

"That's not the way we do it here"

"You could have done better"

Be aware that the use of coercive power will generally result in compliance and only rarely in full commitment. It may also result in resentment and opposition.

	Mostly	Sometimes	Rarely	Comfortable Y/N
I make it clear what standards are required				
I respond to slips from good standards promptly and consistently				
I ensure I have the full facts before using reprimands				
Whenever possible I give warnings in private				
I try to help the person improve on their performance				
I ensure credibility by following up on warnings				
I find out (and reward) what people are doing right				

Handout 3.10: Using expert power

The possession of knowledge, skills or expertise, especially if it is rare and valued, can confer much power on the holder. People who know the best way to perform a procedure or deal with a particular issue and who are up to date with professional developments will have more power than those who do not.

This knowledge must be relevant to the work situation and the influence it confers will be limited to this area of expertise.

It may be necessary to demonstrate that this expertise is both important and not easily available from other sources.

	Mostly	Sometimes	Rarely	Comfortable Y/N
I can give reasons for my requests and explain why they will be useful				
I give these reasons without haranguing or lecturing other people				
I do not overstep the limits of my expertise				
I admit the limits of my expertise and do not try to bluff				
I am aware that other people may have some knowledge of my field and will listen to their contributions				
I stay up to date with developments in my field				

Handout 3.11: Using referent power

This stems from people's desire to please or emulate a person who they admire and respect and who they feel is 'on their side'. The reasons for this might be a recognition of their clinical excellence, their high standards or their concern for their patients and staff. All clinical leaders will possess some of these qualities to some degree. Not everybody can be Florence Nightingale but we can all aim to stimulate respect and loyalty from our teams. Naturally, referent power may be totally independent of formal position and reward or coercive power. You may feel this does not apply to you, that your team take no notice of you. In fact, they will be watching you all the time. More than any other kind of power, referent power elicits commitment rather than mere compliance.

	Mostly	Sometimes	Rarely	Comfortable Y/N
I show concern for my team and support them				
I regard my team positively				
I am sincere in my praise for them				
I act with integrity (truthfulness, consistent values, keeping promises)				
I act as a role model for my team and lead by example				
I understand their values and support them in espousing them				

Handout 4.1: Supporting confidence and competence

1. In the table below, write some ways of supporting your team's confidence and competence *that you are already practising*.

CONFIDENCE	COMPETENCE

2. In the table below, write some ways of supporting your team's confidence and competence *that you will try in the future.*

CONFIDENCE	COMPETENCE

3. In the table below, write some ways of crushing your team's sense of confidence and competence *that you will avoid!*

CONFIDENCE	COMPETENCE

Handout 4.2: Supporting values and meaningfulness

1. In the table below, write some ways of supporting your team's values and sense of meaningfulness *that you already practise.*

2. Below fill in some ways of supporting your team's values and sense of meaningfulness *that you will try in the future.*

3. Below fill in some ways of crushing your team's confidence and competence *that you will avoid!*

Handout 4.3: Supporting a feeling of belongingness

Think back to a time and a place where you felt as if you belonged to a group (it does not have to be a work situation). Below, please write down some of the important things that other people in that group said and did that helped you feel this way.

Think back to a time and a place where you felt as if you did *not* fit in with a group (it does not have to be a work situation). Below, please write down some of the important things that other people in that group said and did that helped you feel this way.

Handout 4.4: Supporting a feeling of belongingness – five top tips

Five top tips for helping new staff to feel that they belong:

1.
2.
3.
4.
5.

Five top tips for helping current and maybe long-serving team members feel that they belong:

1.
2.
3.
4.
5.

Handout 5.1: Our project

Over the next few weeks you will be committing to work on a small project with a team of colleagues.

Guidelines

The project will:

▶ be an exercise in good care

▶ help you demonstrate and grow your Confidence, Competence, Values, Use of Authority and ability to Motivate Others

The project will have modest aims. It may be part of a larger project or entire in itself. It may relate either to patients/residents or to staff, or both.

When considering a project you should think about:

▶ What are your team's strengths?

▶ What does your workplace need?

TITLE

LOCATION

RATIONALE

BACKGROUND

GOAL

STEPS

TIMELINE

How will your project demonstrate the importance of these parts of the Good Care Leadership course?

Confidence and Competence

Values

Use of Authority

Motivating Others

Handout 5.2: A worked example project

TITLE: **Welcoming new staff to Oak Ward**

RATIONALE:

When new qualified staff of any discipline join us, it is clear that they sometimes have difficulty finding their feet. Not only is there a mix of patients with complex clinical conditions but we are a busy multi-disciplinary team. It can be difficult to know what their role is, how decisions are made, how to make their views known and how to make the best of the unique set of skills, knowledge and high standards that they bring with them.

BACKGROUND

There is a relatively high rate of loss of newer qualified staff on Oak Ward. Exit interviews with leavers have shown that new staff often said they felt they did not 'fit in' with the longer serving group.

GOAL

To produce a brief multi-media guide to "How to be a Frontline Leader" using the material from this "Good Care Leadership" course, adapted to the specific needs of Oak Ward.

STEPS

1. Brainstorm with workgroup (who are all current Oak Ward staff) what they felt was good and what was lacking from their induction.

2. Briefly interview all other qualified staff on Oak Ward for their opinions on what they felt was good and what was lacking from their induction.

3. Same interviews with trainees on Oak Ward.

4. Ask other wards in the hospital for their induction procedures.

5. Quick internet and literature search for induction procedures.

6. Meet to collate information from interviews, searches and from the "Good Care Leadership" course. Allocate responsibilities for producing material for the Guide.

7. Writing or recording of allocated responsibilities.

   eg: Staff 1: Write "How to be in charge"

   Staff 2: Video "Growing in confidence"

   Staff 3: Write "You need to know" crib sheets on falls and infection control

   Staff 4: Write "Our vision, your values"

   Staff 5: Video "Tips for motivating your team"

8. Collate literature and videos. Edit and send to secretarial staff for professional formatting.

9. Pilot the guide with new staff on Oak Ward, obtain feedback.

10. Refine the guide as required in the light of feedback.

11. Present to management.

TIMELINE

Feb 26	Step 1
Feb 27–March 5	Steps 2–5
March 5	Step 6
March 6–March 19	Step 7
March 19	Step 8
March 26–April 3	Step 9
April 3–April 10	Step 10
April 12	Step 11

RESOURCES

▶ Support needed from Matron and her line manager

▶ Time required for meetings, interviewing staff, internet searches, writing and recording videos. To be negotiated with management

▶ Videos can be shot on smartphones. Liaise with IT about uploading to Trust system

▶ Secretarial time for professional formatting of document. To be negotiated with management

CONSTRAINTS

▶ Insufficient time available

▶ Allocated time risks being eroded by unforeseen events

▶ Lack of cooperation from other Oak Ward staff

RESPONSIBILITIES

Step 1 Whole group

Steps 2 and 3 Sandra and Alison

Step 4 Brian

Step 5 Ruth

Step 6 Whole group

Step 7 To be decided upon later

Step 8 Sandra and Alison

Step 9 Brian and Ruth

Step 10 Brian

Step 11 Whole group

How will your project demonstrate the importance of these parts of the Good Care Leadership course?

Confidence and Competence

None of the group have any experience in writing this sort of guide, so it will be a learning experience that they believe they can cope with.

This is an opportunity to learn about developing a small video teaching resource. One of us knows all about videos on phones and will teach the others.

Presenting the project will be a challenge, but we will manage okay.

Values

We really believe it is important to welcome new staff and help them feel at home. For themselves and for the smooth running of the ward. This is important.

▶ It is important to show that we care about our new colleagues

▶ It is fair that new staff should be supported and treated equally

▶ We want to show Oak Ward is a friendly and respectful place to work

▶ This is a new venture for us and give us a chance to grow

Use of authority

Expert power – having been on this course we can justify taking people's time for interviews and request their cooperation.

Legitimate power – as qualified nurses backed up by our managers we can request IT support and secretarial support.

Reward power – we will be sincerely grateful to others for their contributions via the interviews.

Referent power – we hope to elicit this by showing our concern for other team members, being good role models and taking action that makes a difference.

Motivating others

By explaining to others the overall significance of the project we hope to motivate them to cooperate with our project.

Powerpoint Slides

The PowerPoint slideshows in this section can be downloaded at
www.pavpub.com/good-care-leadership-resources

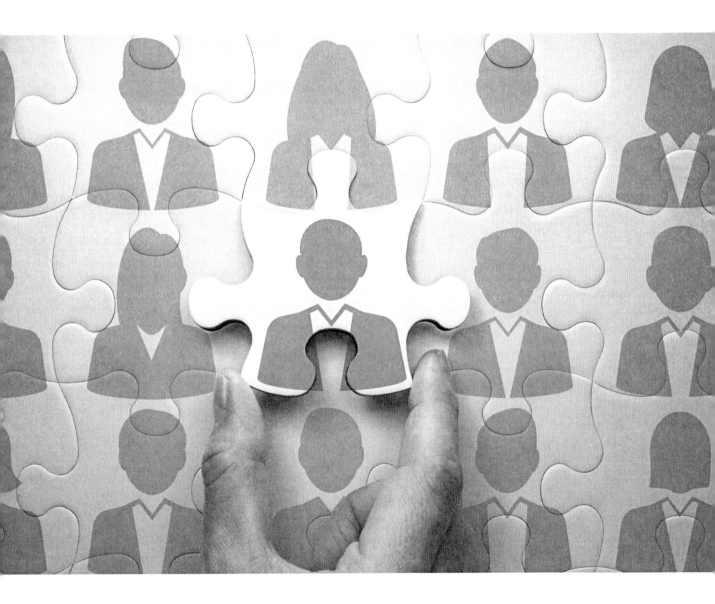

Session 1

Session 1: Confidence and Competence

Welcome

Session 1: Confidence and Competence

Programme

Activity	Time required
Introduction to the session	10 mins
Introduction to confidence	20 mins
Exercise 1.1: When I am more or less confident	30 mins
Exercise 1.2: My career achievements so far	20 mins
Exercise 1.3: Three challenges faced	20 mins
Exercise 1.4: A good leader	30 mins
Exercise 1.5: How am I so wonderful?	40 mins
Session summary	10 mins

Session 1: Confidence and Competence

Four components of good care leadership

1. Confidence and competence
2. Values
3. Use of authority
4. Motivating others

Session 1: Confidence and Competence

Ways of viewing confidence 1

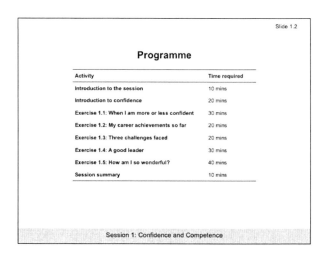

Session 1: Confidence and Competence

Ways of viewing confidence 2

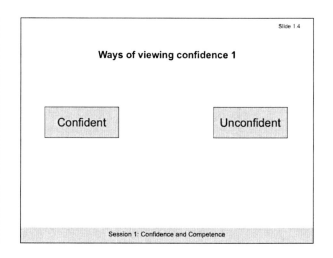

Session 1: Confidence and Competence

False confidence and true confidence

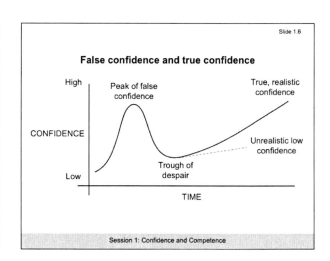

Session 1: Confidence and Competence

Discuss a time I was…

Feeling confident
and
what factors influenced this*?

Feeling unconfident
and
what factors influenced this?

*Hint: These could include: the weather; people around you; how you woke up that morning; something you had been told, or you had read; a 'role model' from work or from elsewhere; bad news; good news; your health; *something* inside you; how well you slept etc.

Session 1: Confidence and Competence

What have I achieved?

Certificates	Special care for a special patient
Promotions	Problems solved
Projects	Challenges accepted
Saving a life	Caring in difficult circumstances
Leading a team	Needs attended to
Making a difference (large or small)	

Session 1: Confidence and Competence

Three challenges

A difficult colleague

A moral dilemma

A difficult decision

A complex task

A complaint

An exam

A 'hopeless' case

What have I learned?

Session 1: Confidence and Competence

Perfect v Useless 1

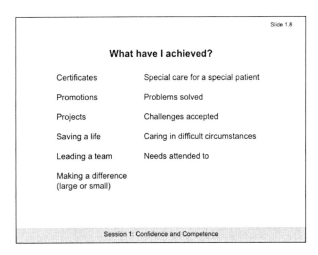

Session 1: Confidence and Competence

Perfect v Useless 2

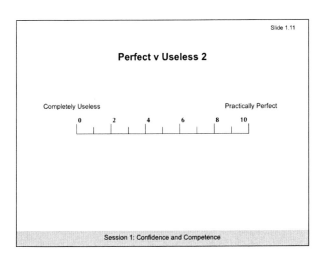

Session 1: Confidence and Competence

Parts of leadership

1. Part of leadership
2. A continuum
3. False confidence
4. Confidence varies
5. Your achievements
6. Three challenges
7. A good leader
8. How am I so wonderful?

EXERCISE 1.1: When I am more or less confident

Four components of good care leadership

1. Confidence in your competence
2. Values
3. Use of authority
4. Motivating others

Session 1: Confidence and Competence

Session 1

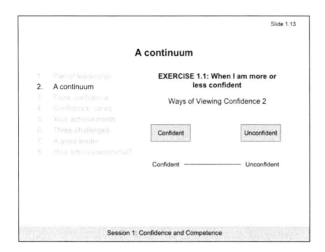

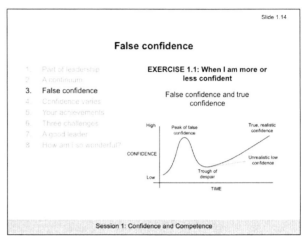

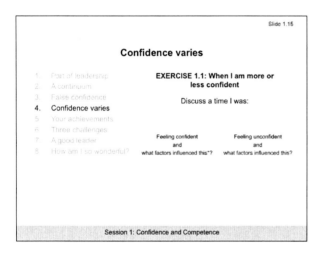

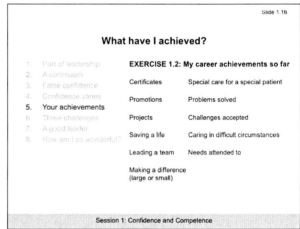

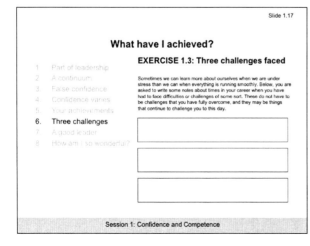

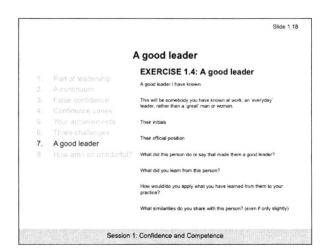

How am I so wonderful?

1. Part of leadership
2. A continuum
3. False confidence
4. Confidence varies
5. Your achievements
6. Three challenges
7. A good leader
8. How am I so wonderful?

Completely Useless   Practically Perfect

0 2 4 6 8 10

Session 1: Confidence and Competence

Session 2

Slide 2.1

Session 2: Personal Values

Welcome

Session 2: Personal Values

Slide 2.2

Programme

Activity	Time required
Introduction to the session	10 mins
Introduction to personal values	20 mins
Exercise 2.1: Writing my own retirement speech	35 mins
Exercise 2.2: Choosing values from the list	35 mins
Exercise 2.3: Realising values in my current work	45 mins
Session summary	15 mins

Session 2: Personal Values

Slide 2.3

Four components of good care leadership

1. Confidence in your competence
2. Values
3. Use of authority
4. Motivating others

Session 2: Personal Values

Slide 2.4

Personal values (1)

- Give meaning to our work
- Are a constant guide for our behaviour – "*Am I on the right track?*" (and the track is not always straight)
- Are associated with strong feelings – including uncomfortable feelings
- Do not need to be reasoned, they are 'just there'
- May never be fully achieved, are constantly in action
- Indicate the direction of travel rather than the destination
- Are personal, but often alike those of others
- Are complementary to professional values

Session 2: Personal Values

Slide 2.5

Personal values (1)

- Give meaning to our work
- **Are a constant guide for our behaviour – "*Am I on the right track?*" (and the track is not always straight)**
- Are associated with strong feelings – including uncomfortable feelings
- Do not need to be reasoned, they are 'just there'
- May never be fully achieved, are constantly in action
- Indicate the direction of travel rather than the destination
- Are personal, but often alike those of others
- Are complementary to professional values

Session 2: Personal Values

Slide 2.6

Personal values (1)

- Give meaning to our work
- Are a constant guide for our behaviour – "*Am I on the right track?*" (and the track is not always straight)
- **Are associated with strong feelings – including uncomfortable feelings**
- Do not need to be reasoned, they are 'just there'
- May never be fully achieved, are constantly in action
- Indicate the direction of travel rather than the destination
- Are personal, but often alike those of others
- Are complementary to professional values

Session 2: Personal Values

Slide 2.7

Personal values (1)

- Give meaning to our work

- Are a constant guide for our behaviour – "*Am I on the right track?*" (and the track is not always straight)

- Are associated with strong feelings – including uncomfortable feelings

- **Do not need to be reasoned, they are 'just there'**

- May never be fully achieved, are constantly in action

- Indicate the direction of travel rather than the destination

- Are personal, but often alike those of others

- Are complementary to professional values

Session 2: Personal Values

Slide 2.8

Personal values (1)

- Give meaning to our work

- Are a constant guide for our behaviour – "*Am I on the right track?*" (and the track is not always straight)

- Are associated with strong feelings – including uncomfortable feelings

- Do not need to be reasoned, they are 'just there'

- **May never be fully achieved, are constantly in action**

- Indicate the direction of travel rather than the destination

- Are personal, but often alike those of others

- Are complementary to professional values

Session 2: Personal Values

Slide 2.9

Personal values (1)

- Give meaning to our work

- Are a constant guide for our behaviour – "*Am I on the right track?*" (and the track is not always straight)

- Are associated with strong feelings – including uncomfortable feelings

- Do not need to be reasoned, they are 'just there'

- May never be fully achieved, are constantly in action

- **Indicate the direction of travel rather than the destination**

- Are personal, but often alike those of others

- Are complementary to professional values

Session 2: Personal Values

Slide 2.10

Personal values (1)

- Give meaning to our work

- Are a constant guide for our behaviour – "*Am I on the right track?*" (and the track is not always straight)

- Are associated with strong feelings – including uncomfortable feelings

- Do not need to be reasoned, they are 'just there'

- May never be fully achieved, are constantly in action

- Indicate the direction of travel rather than the destination

- **Are personal, but often alike those of others**

- Are complementary to professional values

Session 2: Personal Values

Slide 2.11

Personal values (1)

- Give meaning to our work

- Are a constant guide for our behaviour – "*Am I on the right track?*" (and the track is not always straight)

- Are associated with strong feelings – including uncomfortable feelings

- Do not need to be reasoned, they are 'just there'

- May never be fully achieved, are constantly in action

- Indicate the direction of travel rather than the destination

- Are personal, but often alike those of others

- **Are complementary to professional values**

Session 2: Personal Values

Slide 2.12

Personal values (2)

- Give meaning to our work

- Are a constant guide for our behaviour – "*Am I on the right track?*" (and the track is not always straight)

- Are associated with strong feelings – including uncomfortable feelings

- Do not need to be reasoned, they are 'just there'

- May never be fully achieved, are constantly in action

- Indicate the direction of travel rather than the destination

- Are personal, but often alike those of others

- Are complementary to professional values

Session 2: Personal Values

Session 2

My retirement speech

Session 2: Personal Values

Examples

Wisdom	Patience	Order	Mindfulness	Independence
Humility	Flexibility	Gratitude	Safety	Forgiveness
Spirituality	Responsibility	Power	Challenge	Encouragement
Adventure	Intimacy	Pleasure	Romance	Connection
Curiosity	Loyalty	Beauty	Skillfulness	Sexuality
Self-control	Self-development	Self-care	Self-awareness	Supportiveness
Respect	Reciprocity	Open mindedness	Fun	Contribution
Thoughtfulness	Tolerance	Assertiveness	Caring	Authenticity
Cooperation	Conformity	Compassion	Equality	Creativity
Excitement	Fairness	Fitness	Freedom	Friendliness
Generosity	Honesty	Justice	Courage	Humour
Sensuality	Love	Knowledge	Kindness	

Session 2: Personal Values

Examples

- If you choose "Caring" as a value

You might write "*I sat with Mrs Smith and held her hand when she was distressed about her delayed discharge. It would have been easy to leave her alone and get on with my next task*".

- If you choose "Challenge" as a value

You might write "*I chose to take the Dementia Friends course as I know little about dementia and needed to stretch myself*".

Session 2: Personal Values

Parts of leadership

		Personal Values
1.	Part of leadership	1. Confidence in your competence
2.	The nature of values	2. Values
3.	Retirement speech	3. Using your authority
4.	List of values	4. Motivating others
5.	Values in action	

Session 2: Personal Values

The nature of values

Personal Values

1.	Part of leadership	• Give meaning to our work
2.	The nature of values	• Are a constant guide for our behaviour – "*Am I on the right track?*" (and the track is not always straight)
3.	Retirement speech	• Are associated with strong feelings – including uncomfortable feelings
4.	List of values	• Do not need to be reasoned, they are 'just there'
5.	Values in action	• May never be fully achieved, are constantly in action
		• Indicate the direction of travel rather than the destination
		• Are personal, but often alike those of others
		• Are complementary to professional values

Session 2: Personal Values

Retirement speech

Personal Values

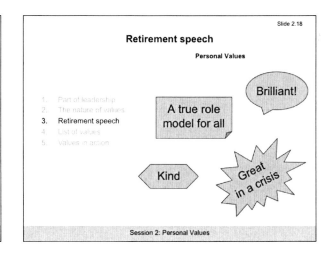

1. Part of leadership
2. The nature of values
3. Retirement speech
4. List of values
5. Values in action

Session 2: Personal Values

Slide 2.19

List of values

Personal Values

1. Part of leadership
2. The nature of values
3. Retirement speech
4. **List of values**
5. Values in action

Wisdom	Patience	Order	Mindful-ness	Independence
Humility	Flexibility	Gratitude	Safety	Forgiveness
Spirituality	Responsibility	Power	Challenge	Encouragement
Adventure	Intimacy	Pleasure	Romance	Connection
Curiosity	Loyalty	Beauty	Skilfulness	Sexuality
Self-control	Self-development	Self-care	Self-awareness	Supportive-ness
Respect	Reciprocity	Open mindedness	Fun	Contribution
Thoughtfulness	Tolerance	Assertive-ness	Caring	Authenticity
Cooperation	Conformity	Compassion	Equality	Creativity
Excitement	Fairness	Fitness	Freedom	Friendliness
Generosity	Honesty	Justice	Courage	Humour
Sensuality	Love	Knowledge	Kindness	

Session 2: Personal Values

Slide 2.20

Values in action

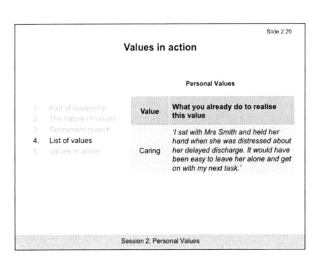

Personal Values

1. Part of leadership
2. The nature of values
3. Retirement speech
4. List of values
5. Values in action

Value	What you already do to realise this value
Caring	*'I sat with Mrs Smith and held her hand when she was distressed about her delayed discharge. It would have been easy to leave her alone and get on with my next task.'*

Session 2: Personal Values

Slide 2.21

Personal values (3)

1. Parts of leadership
2. The nature of values
3. Retirement speech
4. List of values
5. Values in action

Session 2: Personal Values

Session 3

Slide 3.1

Session 3: Use of authority

Welcome

Slide 3.2

Programme

Activity	Time required
Introduction to the session	10 mins
Introduction to the necessity of using your authority	10 mins
Introduction to the five types of power	30 mins
Exercise 3.1: Case study	30 mins
Exercise 3.2: Using power appropriately	45 mins
Exercise 3.3: Feeling comfortable with each of these types of power	40 mins
Challenges in the use of power	10 mins
Session summary	10 mins

Slide 3.3

Four components of good care leadership

1. Confidence in your competence
2. Values
3. Use of authority
4. Motivating others

Slide 3.4

Ward culture

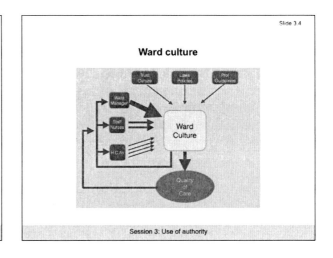

Slide 3.5

Culture change

"On Sunday the 20th of February a different sister was in charge, and the ward felt like a different place. Bells were answered promptly, staff voices seemed lower and the contact with patients felt so much better. Having sat on the ward for four days I observed that this particular nurse's skills at running a ward were exceptional. The ward was a better place when she was around."

Patients Association, 2011, p17

Patients' Association (2011) 'We've been listening, have you been learning?'. Harrow: Patients' Association.

Slide 3.6

The power of the individual

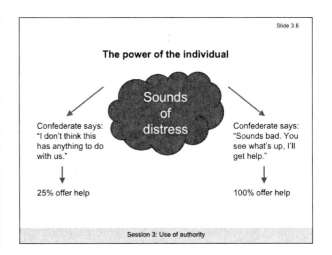

Legitimate/positional power

- Comes with your rank or position of formal authority
- Explicitly stated
- Backed up by the organisation
- Generally accepted
- Extent is defined and limited
- May be challenged if contrary to basic values/principles
- May be indirectly challenged by delay, obstruction or disobedience

Session 3: Use of authority

Using legitimate/positional power

- Respectful and polite requests
- Give reasons for requests
- Requests are clear – written if necessary
- Follow proper channels
- Verify compliance
- Insist on compliance, as appropriate

Session 3: Use of authority

Reward power

- Comes with people knowing you control important rewards
- BUT often you control few material rewards
- Some less tangible rewards – eg training, references

Social rewards

"That was a difficult job done well, thank you"

"Excellent"

"Very professional"

Session 3: Use of authority

Using reward power

- Be fair and ethical. No favourites
- Rewards linked to specific actions
- Rewards are valued
- Praise is appropriate to the individual
- You look out for good work
- Praise more than criticise
- Genuine

Session 3: Use of authority

Coercive power

- Threat of or actual punishment
- Officially sanctioned by formal procedures

Also

- Informal indications of disapproval
- From a frown to a full 'dressing down'
- Gains compliance rather than commitment

Session 3: Use of authority

Using coercive power

- Standards and requirements are clear and well known
- Respond swiftly to lapses
- Criticise the behaviour not the person
- Reprimand in private if possible
- Best used sparingly
- Show how to improve performance
- Follow up on warnings

Session 3: Use of authority

Session 3

Expert power

- Knowledge, skills or expertise
- Most powerful if it is rare
- Must be relevant to the work situation
- Expertise may need to be demonstrated
- Is limited to the area of expertise

Session 3: Use of authority

Using expert power

- Not automatic – may need to be established
- Know your stuff. Stay up to date
- Speak confidently, but do not bluff
- Do not lecture
- Acknowledge others' knowledge and opinions
- Admit the limits of your expertise

Session 3: Use of authority

Referent power

- Personal and non-formal
- Based on respect or admiration
- Being a high standard role model
- Florence Nightingale ☑ David Attenborough ☑
- ALSO Nurse Jones ☑ Sister Green ☑ Matron Smith ☑
- Gains commitment rather than compliance

Session 3: Use of authority

Using referent power

- Showing concern for your team
- Regarding them positively and showing it
- Behaving with integrity, reflecting your values
- Being a consistent role model
- Persisting in all this over time
- Action speaks louder than words

Session 3: Use of authority

Moral challenges

- Temptation of personal gain
- Temptation to harm others
- Avoiding injustice
- Rising to the challenge

Session 3: Use of authority

Using your authority

1. Part of Leadership
2. The influence of the individual
3. The power of the individual
4. Five types of power
5. A case study
6. Using your power appropriately
7. Feeling comfortable using power
8. Moral challenges of leadership

- Confidence and competence
- Values
- Use of authority
- Motivating others

Session 3: Use of authority

Slide 3.19

Using your authority

1. Part of Leadership
2. **The influence of the individual**
3. The power of the individual
4. Five types of power
5. A case study
6. Using your power appropriately
7. Feeling comfortable using power
8. Moral challenges of leadership

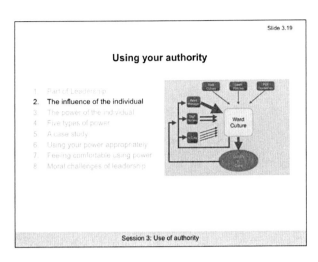

Session 3: Use of authority

Slide 3.20

Using your authority

1. Part of Leadership
2. The influence of the individual
3. **The power of the individual**
4. Five types of power
5. A case study
6. Using your power appropriately
7. Feeling comfortable using power
8. Moral challenges of leadership

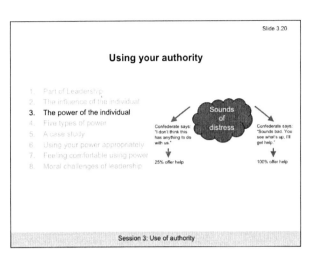

Session 3: Use of authority

Slide 3.21

Using your authority

1. Part of Leadership
2. The influence of the individual
3. The power of the individual
4. **Five types of power**
5. A case study
6. Using your power appropriately
7. Feeling comfortable using power
8. Moral challenges of leadership

1. Legitimate power
2. Reward power
3. Coercive power
4. Expert power
5. Referent power

Session 3: Use of authority

Slide 3.22

Using your authority

1. Part of Leadership
2. The influence of the individual
3. The power of the individual
4. Five types of power
5. **A case study**
6. Using your power appropriately
7. Feeling comfortable using power
8. Moral challenges of leadership

"I believe that giving praise to people for working hard and doing well *is the right thing to do*"

Session 3: Use of authority

Slide 3.23

Using your authority

1. Part of Leadership
2. The influence of the individual
3. The power of the individual
4. Five types of power
5. A case study
6. **Using your power appropriately**
7. Feeling comfortable using power
8. Moral challenges of leadership

Examples
Examples
Examples

Session 3: Use of authority

Slide 3.24

Using your authority

1. Part of Leadership
2. The influence of the individual
3. The power of the individual
4. Five types of power
5. A case study
6. Using your power appropriately
7. **Feeling comfortable using power**
8. Moral challenges of leadership

Comfortable Y/N

Legitimate power
Reward power
Coercive power
Expert power
Referent power

Session 3: Use of authority

Session 3

Slide 3.25

Using your authority

1. Part of Leadership
2. The influence of the individual
3. The power of the individual
4. Five types of power
5. A case study
6. Using your power appropriately
7. Feeling comfortable using power
8. **Moral challenges of leadership**

- Temptation of personal gain
- Temptation to harm others
- Avoiding injustice
- Rising to the challenge

Session 3: Use of authority

Session 4

Session 4: Motivating others

Welcome

Session 4: Motivating others

Programme

Activity	Time required
Introduction to the session	10 mins
Introduction to junk and wholesome motivation	20 mins
Exercise 4.1: Supporting confidence and competence	40 mins
Exercise 4.2: Supporting values and meaning	40 mins
Exercise 4.3: Supporting 'belongingness'	40 mins
Session summary	15 mins

Session 4: Motivating others

Four components of good care leadership

1. Confidence in your competence
2. Values
3. Use of authority
4. Motivating others

Session 4: Motivating others

Complete lack of motivation

"I'm wasting my time in this job"

"This job is not worth putting any energy in to"

"This is a pointless job"

Session 4: Motivating others

Junk food motivation (1)

Carrots and sticks

Limited use

Compliance, not commitment

Unintended consequences

- Demotivation

- Gaming

"I just do it for the pay"

"I risk losing my job if I don't work hard enough"

Session 4: Motivating others

Junk food motivation (2)

Inner critic

- Often concerned with others' rules or expectations

- Uncomfortable, fraught with guilt, shame and anxiety

- Can lead to rigidity and avoidance

"I have to prove myself"

"I would be ashamed of myself if I didn't do a good job"

"I MUST do a perfect job, otherwise I am a total failure"

"What's wrong with me? I SHOULD be able to do better!"

Session 4: Motivating others

Session 4

Slide 4.7

Wholesome motivation (1)

- Reflects one's identity
- Unforced, it springs from within
- Feels comfortable and satisfying

"This job is significant to me"

"This is the kind of person that I am"

"My job is fun" or "My job is interesting"

Session 4: Motivating others

Slide 4.8

Wholesome motivation (2)

Unsurprisingly…

- You cannot MAKE somebody have this high-quality wholesome motivation
- You can only support them to find it

Session 4: Motivating others

Slide 4.9

Three components of wholesome motivation (1)

1. **Confidence and Competence**
2. Values and meaningfulness
3. Belonging

Session 4: Motivating others

Slide 4.10

Confidence and competence

- Achievements
- Challenges
- Role model, a good leader
- Why am I so fabulous? 0–10

Session 4: Motivating others

Slide 4.11

Supporting confidence and competence

- What have people said to you that boosted your confidence?
- Past or present, how have other leaders or managers helped you grow your confidence and competence?
- What are you already doing to grow you team's competence?
- In an ideal situation what would you like to do to support your team's confidence and competence?

Session 4: Motivating others

Slide 4.12

Three components of wholesome motivation (2)

1. Confidence and Competence
2. **Values and meaningfulness**
3. Belonging

Session 4: Motivating others

Values

- Writing my retirement speech
- Choosing values from a list
- How values are realised in day to day work

Supporting values and meaningfulness

- What have people said that demonstrated the value of your work?
- Have others helped you to see how your work fits in with the broader values of your work organisation?
- What are you already doing to make it clear to your team that their work makes a contribution?
- What can you do or say to help people persist with the boring or unpleasant aspects of their job?

Three components of wholesome motivation (3)

1. Confidence and Competence
2. Values and meaningfulness
3. **Belonging**

Belongingness

Wholesome motivation (commitment) is strongly enhanced by:

- Verbal praise
- Referent power
- Sharing expert power

Four components of good care leadership

1. Confidence in your competence
2. Values
3. Use of authority
4. Motivating others

Three aspects of motivation

Lack of motivation

Junk motivation
- Carrots and sticks
- Inner critic

Wholesome motivation
- Meaning in work
- Work reflects values
- Enjoyable or challenging work

Session 4

Three components of wholesome motivation (4)

1. Confidence and Competence

2. Values and meaningfulness

3. Belonging

Session 4: Motivating others

Session 5

Session 5: Project – Putting It Into Practice

Welcome

Session 5: Putting it into practice

Programme

Activity	Time required
Welcome	10 mins
Introduction to projects	20 mins
Writing project plans	1 hour 20 mins
Presenting project plans	40 mins

Session 5: Putting it into practice

Your project will...

- Be an exercise in good care
- Help grow your confidence and competence
- Express or realise your values
- Use your authority
- Help to motivate others in your team

Session 5: Putting it into practice

Your project may...

- Have modest aims
- Relate to either patients or residents or staff
- Be part of a larger project
- Be entire of itself

Session 5: Putting it into practice

When thinking about a project... (1)

- What are team's strengths?
- What does your workplace need?

Session 5: Putting it into practice

When thinking about a project... (2)

- What frustrates you at work?
- What do patients or staff complain about?
- What looks like outdated practice?

or

- If a real hotshot was employed in your place or work, took a look around and saw what was happening, what would she do?

Session 5: Putting it into practice

Session 5

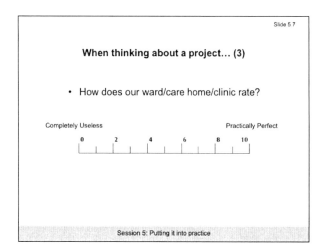

GOOD CARE LEADERSHIP

Certificate of achievement

This is to certify that

....

has attended training on

Good Care Leadership

and covered the following learning outcomes:

1. List and define the four components of frontline leadership and their importance in assuring high quality care

2. Understand and articulate their personal strengths and needs on each of these four components

3. Be able to describe how individuals may influence and lead in their work team

4. Demonstrate the ability to influence their workplace using the four components of frontline leadership

Signed:..

Date:..

Title:..

CPD CERTIFIED
The CPD Certification Service

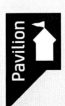

Pavilion

Other titles from Pavilion Publishing

For more information about any of the titles listed here, or to order your copies, go to www.pavpub.com

Staff Supervision in Social Care: Making a real difference for staff and service users

By Tony Morrison

This third edition of the best selling Staff Supervision in Social Care offers essential new material, as well as updating the existing core material covering the fundamentals of good supervision, group supervision and the emotional impact of the work.

This edition extends the understanding and application of the critical links between supervision, the quality of frontline practice and service user outcomes. Increased emphasis is placed on the role of emotional intelligence as crucial to both the quality of supervision and the quality of practice. There is an expanded description of what happens when workers get stuck, exploring the dynamic relationship between the external environment, the supervisee's performance and the internal world of the supervisee. The contribution of the attachment theory to these situations is presented and strategies for addressing such situations are offered. In line with previous editions the manual, it contains a wealth of information, research, practical frameworks, action learning exercises and supervision tools.

It will appeal to both experienced and new supervisors across the social and health care spectrum, both in the UK and internationally.

Professionals within the social care sector are required to undertake Continuous Professional Development (CPD) by the Health and Care Professions Council (HCPC). Those who use this resource will be able to gain CPD points.

Developing and Supporting Effective Staff Supervision. A training pack and reader

By Jane Wonnacott

The *Developing and Supporting Effective Staff Supervision* training pack focuses on training supervisors to deliver one-to-one supervision. Its flexible structure enables trainers to design their own bespoke training programmes. Through group and pair work, participants are actively encouraged to examine and explore their own practice and work together to extend their thinking and improve their skills as supervisors. This pack goes beyond merely teaching theory and actively encourages professional reflection and development.

The training sessions cover: the 4x4x4 model of supervision, the supervision cycle, the impact of emotions, working positively with anxiety, developing and reviewing the supervision agreement and relationship, the blocked cycle, improving practice, and more. This training pack accompanies the *Developing and Supporting Effective Staff Supervision reader* and is for use by experienced trainers who are well grounded in supervision practice and theory.

Professionals within the social care sector are required to undertake Continuous Professional Development (CPD) by the Health and Care Professions Council (HCPC). Those who use this resource will be able to gain CPD points.

Developing and Supporting Effective Staff Supervision. A reader

By Jane Wonnacott

Developing and Supporting Effective Staff Supervision draws on the core concepts in Tony Morrison's *Staff Supervision in Social Care* (Pavilion, 2005) and demonstrates how they can be used to train staff to deliver sound and effective supervision that makes a real difference to service users.

The author of this pack, Jane Wonnacott, was a close colleague of Tony Morrison and worked with him at In-Trac Training and Consultancy Ltd. This reader accompanies the training pack of the same name and is for use by experienced trainers who are well grounded in supervision practice and theory. The reader gives further detail on supervision theory and provides a good source of preparatory material.

While the reader aims to draw out the main building blocks of the supervision model outlined in Staff Supervision in Social Care (Pavilion, 2005), as well as the more recent developments of this the approach, it is not meant to be a 'dumbing down' or an over-simplification of the issues. The underpinning belief throughout the reader is that working with human relationships is complex and demanding and cannot be packaged neatly into a one-size-fits-all prescribed way of responding.

The supervision model and accompanying tools have always been designed to enable practitioners to respond to the individual nature of the issues they are working with and create the a reflective space for exploring challenging issues and ideas, using the knowledge generated through the process to inform both front line practice and the strategic direction of the organisation.

The joy of Morrison's approach has always been the way in which it takes complex ideas, makes them accessible to a wide audience and alongside this gives people tools to help them in their day-to-day practice. This publication aims to continue this approach by reminding readers of core aspects of the model which, if implemented, will provide the foundations for an approach to supervision that makes a real difference to those using social care and health services.

Professionals within the social care sector are required to undertake Continuous Professional Development (CPD) by the Health and Care Professions Council (HCPC). Those who use this resource will be able to gain CPD points.

The Restorative Resilience Model of Supervision. An organisational training manual and reader

By Dr Sonya Wallbank

The Restorative Resilience Model of Supervision: An organisational training manual for building resilience to workplace stress in health and social care professionals is a training pack and accompanying reader that is based on the model of restorative resilience supervision.

Restorative resilience supervision was first developed in response to the emotional demands of midwives, doctors and nurses caring for families who had experienced miscarriage and stillbirth. The programme was designed to support professionals to process their workplace experiences and support them to build resilience levels to ensure they had future coping strategies beyond the initial life of the supervision sessions.

This resource allows an organisation to cascade the restorative resilience approach throughout their staff, initially 'training a trainer', who can then pass the knowledge on to any number of supervisors. It includes full step-by-step instructions for both phases of this training, and a CD-ROM supplying all the handouts and PowerPoints needed to run the training. It also includes several video clips of **Restorative Resilience in action**, modelled by the author, Sonya Wallbank, to demonstrate what good practice should look like.

The reader gives an in-depth understanding of the theoretical principles and research background to the approach, and explores how to put the approach into action on an individual level. In combination with the training pack, this can be used to further the knowledge of all those learning about the approach, both the trainers and the eventual supervisors.

Working with Adults: Values into practice

By Sue Thompson and Jackie Robinson

The importance of child-centred practice as a key part of the value base of working with children and young people is well established. But what about working with adults? How do values make a positive difference? By providing a sound base of understanding and best practice, the authors give trainers and tutors an excellent tool for promoting learning in this area. Topics include promoting dignity – what it means in practice, working in partnerships with service users and carers, legal and moral issues, listening skills, rights and risks, assessment and partnership, continuing professional development and staff care, discrimination and oppression, language sensitivity and workplace culture.

Developing Leadership

By Neil Thompson and Peter Gilbert

Leadership has been a hot topic for some time now, but unfortunately it is subject to a number of common misunderstandings and oversimplifications. In *Developing Leadership*, the authors enable you to benefit from their experience and expertise in clearing away the misunderstandings and helping participants to get to grips with what leadership is really all about. Topics include understanding leadership, styles of leadership, personal and professional values, creating an effective culture, self-awareness, motivation and obstacles to leadership.

The quality of leadership is often the key difference between organisational success and failure and between an organisation being a positive, energising place to work and a negative, stressful environment. Written by two people with a great deal of experience of both serving as leaders and offering training on the subject, this resource has a great deal to offer individuals and organisations committed to developing genuine leadership as a foundation for establishing and maintaining effective and humane workplaces.

Developing this training manual enabled Peter Gilbert to bring together a number of themes around leadership which he had been interested in and engaged with over a number of years – in particular, a holistic approach to leadership.

Reflective Supervision

By Neil Thompson and Peter Gilbert

The supervision of staff is an essential part of effective people management. The quality of supervision can be the difference between acceptable and unacceptable practice at one level and between good and excellent practice at another. *Reflective*

Supervision offers an excellent grounding in the understanding and practice of reflective supervision. Topics include setting the context, promoting anti-discriminatory practice, preparing for supervision, making supervision work, developing reflective practice, recording, giving feedback, providing support, managing poor performance, mediating and trouble shooting.

Promoting Equality, Valuing Diversity

By Neil Thompson

The challenge of developing forms of practice that are effective in tackling discrimination and oppression remains a major one. In *Promoting Equality, Valuing Diversity*, internationally renowned author Dr Neil Thompson explores a wide range of issues relating to equality and diversity. Topics include the case for equality and diversity, understanding and challenging discrimination in relation to age, race and ethnicity, gender, sexual orientation, disability and religion.

Tackling Bullying and Harassment in the Workplace

By Neil Thompson

Bullying and harassment continue to be major problems in the modern workplace. This manual provides the basis for the training of staff and managers to recognise, respond to and prevent bullying and harassment. Topics include understanding bullying and harassment, the law, resisting the bully, positive leadership, sexual, racial and other forms of harassment, dangerous organisations, policy and practice, taking staff care seriously.

She'll be Alright. A story-based approach to exploring issues of hidden neglect in care homes

By Alex Matthews

She'll Be Alright is a series of short episodes showing neglect in an English nursing home. These are the stories of people who can no longer speak for themselves which invite the reader to access the world of care as it unfolds behind closed doors. The characters' real names have been changed and the events have been slightly altered in order to create works of fiction, but the stories presented here are true in essence and have not been exaggerated in any respect.

She'll be Alright has been written so that people can use this guide in order to gain valuable insights into a world that is usually only visible to those involved with neglect cases. The case studies in *She'll Be Alright* give readers access to material specially designed for learning and self-development, cross-referenced to the relevant legislation, and complemented with reflection and discussion questions.

This training and self-study guide explores the following topics:

▶ Safeguarding residents in nursing and care homes, in particular dementia service users

▶ Supporting nursing and care home staff and dementia workers

▶ Improving management and supervision within residential settings

▶ End of life care and palliative care for dementia.

▶ How to apply the Fundamental Care Standards and the Code of Conduct for Healthcare Support Workers and Adult Social Care Workers in England in order to identify hidden neglect and make a disclosure.

Person-centred Lifestyles for People with Intellectual Disabilities. Transforming attitudes, services and practice

By Hilary Brown and Jan Alcoe

Person-centred Lifestyles for People with Intellectual Disabilities is a simple but powerful staff and service development exercise that provides a vital stimulus to exploring and evaluating attitudes, services and practice in relation to people with intellectual disabilities and the quality of lives they are enabled to lead.